D1319742

The Effects of Estrogen
on Brain Function

The Effects of Estrogen on Brain Function

Edited by

N A T A L I E L. R A S G O N , M.D., Ph.D.
Associate Professor of Psychiatry and
of Obstetrics and Gynecology
Director, Behavioral Neuroendocrinology Program
and Women's Wellness Program
Department of Psychiatry and Behavioral Sciences
Stanford University School of Medicine
Stanford, California

The Johns Hopkins University Press
Baltimore

© 2006 The Johns Hopkins University Press
All rights reserved. Published 2006
Printed in the United States of America on acid-free paper

2   4   6   8   9   7   5   3   1

The Johns Hopkins University Press
2715 North Charles Street
Baltimore, Maryland 21218-4363
www.press.jhu.edu

Peter J. Schmidt contributed to chapter 6 as a work of the U.S. government.

Library of Congress Cataloging-in-Publication Data
The effects of estrogen on brain function / edited by Natalie L. Rasgon.
p. ; cm.
Includes bibliographical references and index.
ISBN 0-8018-8282-6 (hardcover : alk. paper)
1. Cognition disorders—Endocrine aspects. 2. Estrogen—Therapeutic use—
Complications. 3. Brain—Effect of drugs on. 4. Menopause—Hormone therapy—
Complications.   I. Rasgon, Natalie L.
[DNLM: 1. Estrogen Replacement Therapy. 2. Estrogens—pharmacology.
3. Central Nervous System—drug effects. 4. Cognition—drug effects. 5. Risk
Assessment.   WP 522 E27 2006]
RC553.C64E44 2006
616.8′0461—dc22   2005019344

ACC Library Services
Austin, Texas

Contents

Contributors

Roberta Diaz Brinton, Ph.D., Professor, Department of Molecular Pharmacology and Toxicology and Program in Neuroscience, Pharmaceutical Sciences Center, University of Southern California, Los Angeles, California

Cheri L. Geist, B.A., Assistant, Division of Biological Imaging, Department of Molecular and Medical Pharmacology, David Geffen School of Medicine, University of California at Los Angeles, California

Robert B. Gibbs, Ph.D., Professor, Department of Pharmaceutical Sciences, University of Pittsburgh School of Pharmacy, Pennsylvania

Eva Hogervorst, Ph.D., Chair of Psychology, Department of Human Sciences, University of Loughborough; Oxford Project to Investigate Memory and Ageing, Department of Pharmacology, University of Oxford, United Kingdom

Pauline M. Maki, Ph.D., Associate Professor, Center for Cognitive Medicine, Departments of Psychiatry and Psychology, Neuropsychiatric Institute, University of Illinois–Chicago, Illinois

Peter J. Schmidt, M.D., Chief, Unit on Reproductive Endocrine Studies, Behavioral Endocrinology Branch, National Institute of Mental Health, Bethesda, Maryland

Daniel H. S. Silverman, M.D., Ph.D., Associate Professor and Head, Neuronuclear Imaging Section; Associate Chief, Division of Biological Imaging, Department of Molecular and Medical Pharmacology, David Geffen School of Medicine, University of California at Los Angeles, California

Katherine E. Williams, M.D., Clinical Research Physician, Behavioral Neuroendocrinology Program, and Women's Wellness Clinic; Co-director Behavioral Neuroendocrinology Program, Department of Psychiatry and Behavioral Sciences, Stanford University School of Medicine, California

Kristine Yaffe, M.D., Departments of Psychiatry, Neurology, and Epidemiology, University of California, San Francisco, and San Francisco VA Medical Center, California

Laurel N. Zappert, M.S., Clinical Research Associate, Behavioral Neuroendocrinology Program, Department of Psychiatry and Behavioral Sciences, Stanford University School of Medicine, California

Liqin Zhao, Ph.D., Research Scientist, Department of Molecular Pharmacology and Toxicology and Program in Neuroscience, Pharmaceutical Sciences Center, University of Southern California, Los Angeles, California

The Effects of Estrogen
on Brain Function

Introduction

NATALIE L. RASGON, M.D., Ph.D.

The use of hormone therapy (HT) has come under considerable scrutiny in recent years, and the implications of past and current HT research for women's health are manifold. Currently, a woman can expect to live nearly one-third of her life in postmenopause, as the average life expectancy for women in the United States has increased to 82 years, while the average age of menopause has remained at 51 years. The issue of risks versus benefits from estrogen use has been discussed for several decades, and despite significant research efforts, the debate continues. For many women and their treating physicians, the decision to initiate or continue HT is based on consideration of individual risk factors, including the risk for stroke, cancer, or Alzheimer disease (AD), and beneficial lifestyle factors, such as a reduction in hot flushes, night sweats, and depression, along with the risks and benefits associated with long-term treatment with a steroid agent. In 1979, the National Institute on Aging convened the Consensus Development Conference on Estrogen Use and Postmenopausal Women to explore the risks and benefits of estrogen use, which were of interest to the 31 million postmenopausal women and their physicians in the United States. Among the topics discussed were the benefits of estrogen therapy (ET) in the treatment of menopausal symptoms and to prevent osteoporosis, the relative risks and benefits of different types of ET, the hazards of estrogen use, and indications for and contraindications to ET (National Institute on Aging, 1979).

At the time of the conference, it was accepted that estrogens were more effective than placebo in decreasing the frequency and severity of vasomotor symptoms, including hot flushes and sweating. Estrogens were also known to be effective in counteracting atrophy of the vaginal epithelium and associated symptoms, including burning, itching, dryness, and pain during intercourse. Whether vasomotor symptoms had a single cause and why some women needed much larger doses than others to control symptoms were questions that still awaited answers. There was general agreement that the decision to initiate therapy should depend on the severity of the symptoms and on the patient's apparent need for relief. It was also generally accepted that the lowest effective dose should be used for the shortest period, as the occurrence of hot flushes naturally decreases over time (National Institute on Aging, 1979).

Controversy existed, however, on several issues, including the use of estrogens to treat mood problems and the effects of estrogen on sleep. In addition, the risks of using various progestins to decrease the occurrence of endometrial hyperplasia and cancer of the endometrium had not been adequately evaluated. One area of general agreement among the participants was that a woman seeking HT should be given as much information as possible about the evidence for the efficacy of estrogens in treating specific menopausal conditions and the risks associated with the use of HT. Further study would be needed to understand the natural course of menopause without HT and to determine alternatives to estrogen use, optimal HT preparations and methods of administration, and the beneficial and adverse effects of HT use (National Institute on Aging, 1979).

In 1992, the American College of Physicians, the American College of Family Medicine, and the U.S. Preventive Services Task Force put their weight behind guidelines that encouraged physicians to prescribe HT for women with or at risk for heart disease and osteoporosis. The data that formed the basis of these guidelines showed that women who took estrogen or a combination of estrogen and progesterone had a 35 to 50 percent reduced risk of heart attack (Vastag, 2002).

As outlined in the summary of a National Institutes of Health (NIH) scientific workshop on menopausal HT, the NIH implemented the Women's Health Initiative (WHI) in the early 1990s to assess the overall benefits and risks of HT and to determine whether long-term HT could prevent coronary heart disease (CHD) in postmenopausal women (Kirschstein, 2003). Women 50 to 79 years of age who had not undergone a hysterectomy were randomly assigned to re-

ceive PremPro (0.625 mg of conjugated equine estrogen plus 2.5 mg of medroxyprogesterone) or placebo. Women who had undergone hysterectomy received Premarin (estrogen alone) or placebo (Kirschstein, 2003). After approximately five years, the PremPro trial was discontinued in July 2002 because
the risks of combination estrogen and progesterone (specifically, increased
rates of CHD, breast cancer, stroke, and pulmonary embolism) were considered to outweigh the benefits (lowered rates of colorectal cancer and hip fracture). The Premarin arm of WHI was discontinued in March 2004 because of
an increased risk for stroke, similar to that in the PremPro arm of the study
(Anderson et al., 2004).

The NIH convened another scientific workshop on menopausal HT in Oc-
tober 2002, with the purpose of discussing the results and reasons for discon-
tinuing the WHI combination estrogen plus progesterone trial to help clini-
cians and their patients better understand the data available on the risks and
benefits of short- and long-term combination HT. Although a number of earlier
epidemiological studies had suggested cardioprotective effects for estrogen,
several systematic evaluations found the opposite. For example, in the Postmenopausal Estrogen/Progestin Interventions (PEPI) trial, the effects of estrogen alone and of estrogen plus progestin on risk factors for CHD were evaluated, and although the results were promising, the investigators could not
directly test whether CHD could be prevented through the use of HT (Writing
Group for the PEPI Trial, 1995). The Heart and Estrogen/Progestin Replacement Study (HERS), a secondary prevention trial of combination estrogen and
progesterone, found indications of early harm, and no benefits for CHD (Hulley
et al., 1998; Kirschstein, 2003).

The National Institute on Aging is continuing to support research on the effects of ET, and this research is based on epidemiological and small clinical
studies that have indicated a decreased risk for cognitive deficits and AD in
women who use ET. Of 24 treatment studies conducted from 1976 to 2001,
6 found positive effects, 11 were equivocal, and 7 showed no effect. Two
studies were discontinued in 2002 because of negative findings: the WHI
Memory Study (WHIMS), which examined all stages of dementia in women
65 years of age or older, and the WHI Study of Cognitive Aging (WHISCA),
which assessed whether HT protects against age-associated memory and cognitive decline in women over the age of 65.

In the WHIMS study, subjects received conjugated equine estrogens with or
without (Premarin-alone arm) medroxyprogesterone acetate (MPA), an agent

that is associated with an increased risk of stroke, breast cancer, and pulmonary embolism. It is possible that both PremPro and Premarin are not optimal choices for therapy, particularly in older women (65 and older). Research to ascertain the varying effects of different HT preparations, routes of administration, and treatment durations on cognitive function is needed.

Assessing and Communicating Risks and Benefits

Although the WHI had previously focused on prevention, and not on quality-of-life or symptom relief benefits, the news media and the general public often do not understand the subtlety of the WHI results, especially the concepts of absolute versus relative risk associated with HT use. For example, although the relative risk for breast cancer among WHI study participants taking estrogen plus progesterone increased 26 percent during the five years of the study, the absolute risk for an individual woman was small. Furthermore, results from the Premarin-alone arm suggested a strong trend toward a decreased breast cancer risk and no negative effect on CHD risk. The issue that should be addressed by patients and their physicians today is disease risk versus the benefits of symptom relief and improved quality of life.

Currently, more than 40 million women are taking HT to relieve menopausal symptoms, and only 20 percent of these women stay on these regimens longer than five years. Both the American College of Obstetricians and Gynecologists and the North American Menopause Society recommend that combination HT be used for the shortest duration consistent with treatment goals and benefits versus risks for individual women, taking into account quality-of-life issues. Alternative delivery methods such as vaginal tablets, vaginal creams, or a vaginal ring can be effective and do not appreciably increase systemic estrogen levels. Few studies, however, have assessed the long-term benefit–risk ratios of these alternatives. The North American Menopause Society stated that the WHI data could not be extrapolated directly to symptomatic perimenopausal women, women experiencing early menopause (40–50 years of age), or those undergoing premature menopause (<40 years of age).

More information is needed about doses, drugs, preparations, administration methods, alternative therapies, and supplements, because there is still confusion about the benefits and risks of HT. This is especially important because no current option offers symptom relief comparable to that of combination HT.

Overview of Chapters

This book reviews available data on basic and clinical aspects of the effects of HT in the central nervous system and outlines a number of questions that need to be addressed in future studies. In chapter 1, Robert Gibbs notes that animal data provide persuasive evidence for the use of either estrogen alone or combination HT to enhance cognitive performance and ameliorate the age-related decline in cognitive function after the loss of ovarian function. The timing of administration is critical, as animal studies suggest that in order for HT to be effective, it must be initiated within a limited period after loss of ovarian function. Gibbs also points out that a majority of randomized clinical trials, including WHIMS, have focused exclusively on the effects of HT in women who are 65 years of age and older, which is beyond the "window of opportunity" to obtain the benefits of HT on cognitive performance. Finally, compared with estrogen alone or the cyclical administration of estrogen and progesterone, long-term simultaneous combination therapy is not beneficial and may have adverse effects on cognitive function, especially basal forebrain cholinergic function. These results are consistent with observational studies and may help explain the differences between the results of these studies and WHIMS. Consequently, in spite of the WHI findings, Gibbs predicts that HT can have a beneficial effect on postmenopausal women, provided that the treatment dose and regimen are appropriate and treatment is initiated at the proper time in the menopausal transition.

In her review of the effects of HT on cognitive function in human studies (chapter 2), Eva Hogervorst argues that no current evidence suggests that treatment with HT for longer than a year prevents cognitive decline in women with or without dementia. The effects of HT appear to be short-lived and reverse after one year in postmenopausal women. For younger women who undergo longer treatment with HT, there is no evidence that these effects are positive.

Additionally, while MPA has negative effects, other progestagens have not been demonstrated to have additional negative effects on cognitive function. As Hogervorst points out, however, these studies on progestagens were of short duration and enrolled young, symptomatic women; it is unclear whether different results might emerge with a longer follow-up. It also remains to be elucidated whether women who have severe vasomotor symptoms or who have undergone surgical menopause can benefit from longer durations of treatment with HT. There is great need for more research in this area, because no alternative treatments are available to reverse cognitive decline in elderly women.

The field of neuroimaging has provided new and critical information on the effects of HT on cerebral metabolism and neurocognitive decline. Before the advent of positron emission tomography (PET), magnetic resonance imaging, and functional magnetic resonance imaging, little was known about the gender-associated effects of gonadal steroids on neuronal function and neurochemistry, and new information about the effects of estrogen on the female brain has been provided by this neuroimaging technology. In chapter 3, Daniel Silverman, Cheri Geist, and Natalie Rasgon provide an overview of PET findings relating to cerebral metabolism and HT, and highlight data showing that patients whose PET patterns were indicative of progressive dementia were 18 times more likely to experience progressive decline than were those with nonprogressive PET patterns. This finding increased the likelihood of a correct diagnosis of progressive dementia by as much as 84 percent. A positive diagnosis based on PET results increased the accuracy of this prediction of cognitive decline to 94 percent, and a negative PET study made it 12 times more likely that the patient would remain cognitively stable. This has great implications for the treatment of progressive dementia, as proper and early diagnosis could help treatment in the future, especially with the new treatment modalities currently being developed and tested.

The effects of HT on mood have received more attention as of late, and our findings, among others, suggest that the use of estrogen in certain groups of women during the postpartum period and the perimenopausal transition can be beneficial. Our review of the data in chapter 4 suggests that (1) women undergoing the menopausal transition who have had prior mood episodes are more likely to have a recurrence during the menopausal transition; (2) a bimodal relationship exists between length of reproductive life and major depressive disorder; (3) treatment with estradiol alone may be effective in the treatment of perimenopausal women with mild depression or dysthymia, but there is no evidence that estradiol alone is effective in older women with major depressive disorder; and (4) estradiol may be effective as an adjunctive treatment to antidepressants in peri- and postmenopausal women with major depressive disorder. These studies are only preliminary, and larger and longer, controlled longitudinal studies are needed to define a population of women who would be likely to respond well to estrogen as a monotherapy or to estrogen augmentation. Furthermore, it is critical to properly identify patients who are vulnerable to new or recurring mood disorders because of changes in estrogen levels, and to define the risks and benefits of ET for these women.

In chapter 5, Roberta Brinton and Liqin Zhao review the preclinical efforts being made to develop effective brain selective estrogen receptor modulators (NeuroSERMs) and discuss the mechanistic understanding of why ET is efficacious in the prevention but not the treatment of AD. Specifically, the authors note that the calcium-dependent mechanisms of estrogen action in neurons underlie the healthy-cell bias for estrogen-inducible proactive neuroprotection against degenerative insults and promotion of morphogenesis in neurons. Research is now being conducted to develop NeuroSERMs that promote the neurotrophic and neuroprotective benefits of estrogen in the brain while not inducing the adverse effects of estrogens. The realization of such efforts to develop proactive defensive therapies could help prevent age-related dementias such as AD.

In chapter 6, Kristine Yaffe, Pauline Maki, and Peter Schmidt review the biological mechanisms that explain the beneficial effects of SERMs on cognition and brain metabolism. Preliminary data point to a reduction in the risk of cognitive decline in patients who are given raloxifene, a finding that underscores the need for further research on raloxifene and other SERMs. Finally, Yaffe and co-authors discuss genetic factors in sex hormone pathways that may affect cognitive decline and the response of patients to endogenous steroids.

REFERENCES

Anderson GL, Limacher M, Assaf AR, et al. 2004. Effects of conjugated equine estrogen in postmenopausal women with hysterectomy: the Women's Health Initiative randomized controlled trial. JAMA 291:1701–12.

Hulley S, Grady D, Bush T, et al., for the Heart and Estrogen/Progestin Replacement Study Research Group. 1998. Randomized trial of estrogen plus progestin for secondary prevention of coronary heart disease in postmenopausal women. JAMA 280: 605–13.

Kirschstein R. 2003. Menopausal hormone therapy: summary of a scientific workshop. Ann Intern Med 138:361–64.

National Institute on Aging. 1979. Consensus Development Conference on Estrogen Use and Postmenopausal Women. Bethesda, Md., September 13–14.

Vastag B. 2002. Hormone replacement therapy falls out of favor with expert committee. JAMA 287:1923–24.

The Writing Group for the PEPI Trial. 1995. Effects of estrogen or estrogen/progestin regimens on heart disease risk factors in postmenopausal women: the Postmenopausal Estrogen/Progestin Interventions (PEPI) trial. JAMA 273:199–208.

CHAPTER ONE

Preclinical Data Relating to Estrogen's Effects on Cognitive Performance

ROBERT B. GIBBS, Ph.D.

The use of gonadal hormone therapy (HT) in peri- and postmenopausal women has become a major public health issue. Within the last hundred years, the average life expectancy of women in the United States has risen beyond 82 years, whereas the average age at which women reach menopause has remained relatively constant at 51 years. In addition to more years of life after menopause, approximately 600,000 hysterectomies are performed each year in the United States (Farquhar and Steiner, 2002), many of which include removal of the ovaries (surgical menopause). In fact, it is estimated that one in every three women in the United States will undergo ovariectomy before the age of 60. As a consequence of both increased longevity and the early induction of menopause, women can now expect to spend nearly one-third of their adult lives in the postmenopausal state.

Never before have women been faced with so many choices for HT or with so much information about the effects of HT on physiology and behavior. For many, the decision to initiate or continue HT is based not only on the immediate benefits of the therapy but also on the risks and benefits of an extended course of treatment. Individual risk factors must now be assessed and weighed against the importance of maintaining lifestyle and the fear of debilitating age-related diseases, such as cancer, stroke, and Alzheimer disease (AD). Unfortunately, the long-term effects of many of the available treatment regimens are still unknown, and there is considerable disagreement over how the vast quantity of information should be interpreted and applied in an individual case.

Data from animal studies indicate that HT can have a multitude of beneficial effects on brain function, including protecting the brain from injury, improving cognitive performance, and preventing or slowing age-related cognitive decline. The results of human trials are less clear, and even the most recent clinical studies have done little to resolve this issue. On the one hand, observational studies suggest that women who use HT after menopause are less likely to develop AD than are nonusers (Henderson, 2000; LeBlanc et al., 2001). In contrast, results of the Women's Health Initiative Memory Study (WHIMS), a randomized, placebo-controlled, clinical trial, showed that women who received HT consisting of conjugated equine estrogens (CEE) plus medroxyprogesterone acetate (MPA) were twice as likely to develop probable dementia over a five-year period as women who received placebo (Shumaker et al., 2003). In addition, women treated with CEE alone showed a greater risk for dementia and global cognitive decline, particularly women with lower cognitive ratings at the initiation of treatment (Espeland et al., 2004; Shumaker et al., 2004). The apparent contradiction in study results, along with recent evidence of an increased risk of stroke, pulmonary embolism, and breast cancer associated with the long-term use of combination therapy, has greatly reduced enthusiasm for HT and its possible benefits with respect to brain aging and cognition (Mulnard et al., 2004).

This chapter reviews the recent animal literature as it pertains to the effects of HT on cognitive performance. Based on this literature, we believe that many of the apparent contradictions can be resolved and that postmenopausal HT can help to prevent age-related cognitive decline in women, if the therapy is initiated around the time of menopause and at a dose and in a regimen appropriate for the brain.

The Effects of Estrogen Therapy on Cognitive Performance

Studies from different laboratories have demonstrated repeatedly that ovariectomized rats that receive estradiol perform better on a variety of cognitive tasks than do ovariectomized controls not given estradiol. The majority of these studies have focused on tests of spatial learning and working memory. Work by Dohanich and co-workers (reviewed in Dohanich, 2002) has shown that treatment with estradiol for at least one week before training enhances acquisition of reinforced alternation and radial arm maze performance by ovariectomized rats. Similar studies have shown enhanced working mem-

ory performance in rats treated with estradiol and tested using standard radial
arm maze, water radial maze, and working memory versions of the Morris
water maze task (Bimonte and Denenberg, 1999; Daniel et al., 1999). Our own
studies have shown estradiol-mediated enhancement in the acquisition of
competency on a delayed matching-to-position T-maze task, a task in which
animals must learn to return to a previously entered arm of a T-maze to receive a food reward (Fig. 1.1). Similar results have been reported in mice,
where the administration of estradiol has been shown to enhance both place
learning and performance on a simplified radial arm maze task (Heikkinen
et al., 2002).

The enhancing effects of estrogen are not limited to spatial tasks or to tasks
involving food reward. For example, studies have shown that estrogens enhance visual object recognition in rats (Birke, 1979; Luine et al., 2003) and
visual place memory in both rats and mice (Li et al., 2004; Luine et al., 2003).
This enhancement was observed when estrogens (estradiol or diethylstilbe-

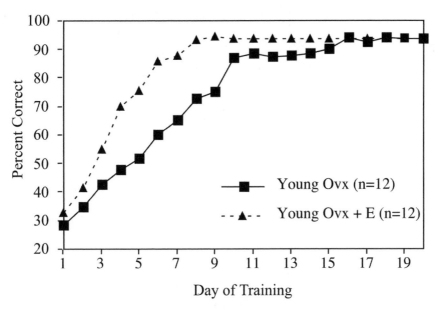

Fig. 1.1 Estradiol enhances the acquisition of a delayed matching-to-position T-maze
task by young ovariectomized rats. Values represent the mean percentage of correct
responses for each group on each day of training.
Source: Gibbs and Gabor, 2003. Reprinted with permission.

strol) were injected shortly before training or immediately after training, but not when they were injected two hours after training (Fig. 1.2). The fact that estrogens were effective when administered immediately *after* training demonstrates an effect on mnemonic processes, such as consolidation or encoding, as opposed to an effect on motivation or performance parameters. In monkeys, estradiol has been shown to modulate visuospatial attention (Voytko, 2002)

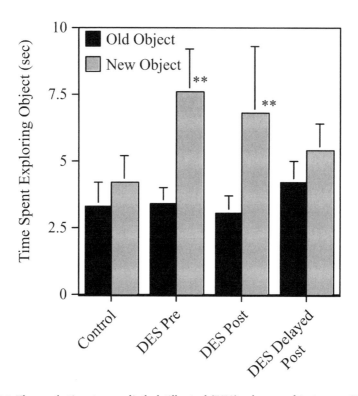

Fig. 1.2 The synthetic estrogen diethylstilbestrol (DES) enhances object recognition in young ovariectomized rats. Animals were exposed to two novel objects during a sample trial and then exposed to one familiar object and one novel object 4 hours later during a recognition trial. Bars indicate time spent exploring the familiar and novel objects during the recognition trial. Treatment groups include vehicle-treated controls and animals that received DES either 30 minutes before (DES Pre), immediately after (DES Post), or 2 hours after (DES Delayed Post) the sample trial. Note that DES increased exploration of the novel object when injected before or immediately after the sample trial but not when injected 2 hours after the sample trial, suggesting an effect on memory consolidation. $^{**}P < 0.01$ relative to time spent with the familiar object. *Source:* Adapted from Luine et al., 2003, © 2003 The Endocrine Society.

and to enhance performance on delayed response and delayed nonmatching-to-sample tasks (Rapp et al., 2003). Collectively, these findings demonstrate that the administration of estrogen can enhance performance on a wide variety of cognitive tasks in both rodents and nonhuman primates.

Hormone therapy does not enhance performance on all tasks, however. For example, the performance of young adult rats on a spatial version of the Morris water maze task was impaired, not enhanced, by elevated levels of estradiol and progesterone (Chesler and Juraska, 2000). In monkeys, estradiol had no effect on the performance of a simple reaction time task (Voytko, 2002) and no effect on an object discrimination task (Rapp et al., 2003). We recently examined learning using a configural association operant conditioning task. Rats were trained to associate simple stimuli such as a stimulus light and stimulus tone with food reward. Simultaneous presentation of the light and tone, however, resulted in no food reward, extinction of the house light, and a "time-out." Animals therefore had to learn to discriminate between positive reinforcement associated with each of the simple stimuli and negative reinforcement associated with combined presentation of the two stimuli. Notably, estradiol had no significant effect on the acquisition of this task (Fig. 1.3), despite the positive effects of estrogen on learning that were detected with other appetitive tasks.

These findings suggest that (1) estrogen treatment enhances cognitive performance within specific cognitive domains and (2) the effects of estrogen treatment on cognitive performance are not due simply to a global effect on nonspecific performance factors, such as motivation and perceptual abilities, because estrogen had no significant effect on tasks with similar motivational and perceptual demands.

In humans, clinical studies performed with surgically menopausal and naturally menopausal women have yielded similar results. Women receiving HT, either estrogen therapy or a combination of estrogen plus progestin therapy, often are reported to perform better on some tasks, but not all tasks, than controls (Sherwin, 2002). Problems arise when attempting to generalize individual results across clinical trials because of inconsistent findings on which cognitive tasks are most affected (Hogervorst et al., 2002; Sherwin, 2002). In two meta-analyses, Hogervorst et al. (2000, 2002) reported small effects of HT on several aspects of cognitive function, such as memory, attention, reaction time speed, and abstract reasoning, although the effects were not always consistent from one study to the next. Another study found positive correlations between total estradiol and testosterone levels and performance on specific sex-sensitive

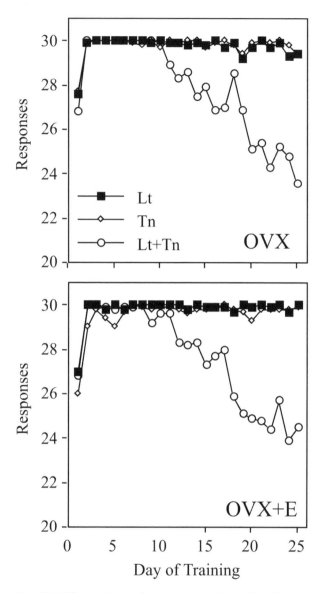

Fig. 1.3 Estradiol did not enhance the acquisition of a configural association negative patterning task by young ovariectomized rats. Values indicate the mean number of responses to the stimulus light (positive association), the stimulus tone (positive association), and simultaneous presentation of the light and tone (negative association) (n = 10/group).

Source: Gibbs and Gabor, 2003. Reprinted with permission.

tests (e.g., verbal list recall, spatial span performance) in older men and women not receiving HT (Hogervorst et al., 2004). These effects were unchanged after controlling for education, sex hormone–binding globulin levels, body mass index, depression, daily alcohol use, and smoking. These findings are consistent with results from animal studies in suggesting that in women, HT can have small but significant positive effects on cognitive performance.

In sum, both animal and human studies consistently indicate that estrogen therapy affects performance on some but not all cognitive tasks, suggesting that estrogen therapy affects performance within specific cognitive domains. Precisely which cognitive domains are affected and to what degree continue to be debated; however, it is clear that estrogen therapy influences cognitive performance and that the effects are not due merely to effects on motivational factors or perceptual abilities.

The Effects of Estrogen Therapy on Age-Related Cognitive Decline

An important question is whether HT can help prevent or reduce age-related cognitive decline. Alzheimer disease, which accounts for the majority of cases of age-related dementia, affects approximately 6 to 10 percent of the population over age 65 (Hendrie, 1998). In the United States, 4 million Americans currently have AD, and it is estimated that by the middle of the twenty-first century, AD will affect 8 to 13 million Americans, most of them women (Brookmeyer et al., 1998).

Animal studies have provided some direct evidence that treatment with either estrogen or estrogen plus progesterone can help to prevent or treat age-related cognitive decline. One study showed that, despite contrary results in young adult mice, treatment of older mice with estradiol produced a dose-related improvement in spatial reference memory (Frick et al., 2002). Another study showed that, in middle-aged rats ovariectomized at 14 months of age, ovarian hormone treatment (including acute estradiol treatment, long-term estradiol treatment, and long-term estradiol plus progesterone treatment) prevented overnight forgetting on a spatial version of the Morris water maze task (Markham et al., 2002). The administration of estradiol has been shown to enhance T-maze learning and behavioral reversal learning (a measure of cognitive flexibility) in Ts65D mice, a mouse model of Down syndrome (Granholm et al., 2002). β-Amyloid production is a hallmark of AD. Estradiol has been shown to protect against the neurotoxic effects of β-amyloid (Marin et al., 2003) and to reduce the generation of β-amyloid by neuroblastoma cells and by primary cultures of rat, mouse, and human embryonic cerebrocortical neurons (Xu et al., 1998), all of which may help to protect against the development of Alzheimer-related dementia.

Our own studies have shown that long-term treatment with either estradiol or a cyclical regimen of estradiol and progesterone can significantly reduce the development of age-related impairment on a delayed matching-to-position T-maze task (Gibbs, 2000b). In this study, rats were ovariectomized at midlife and then received either continuous low-level estradiol treatment beginning immediately or 3 months following ovariectomy, or weekly administration of estradiol (on Monday) and progesterone (on Wednesday) beginning 3 months or 10 months following ovariectomy. Controls received vehicle instead of hormone treatment. All animals were tested at an advanced age (23–25 months) on a delayed matching-to-position T-maze task. The results showed that animals that received either estradiol alone or weekly administration of estradiol and progesterone initiated within three months after ovariectomy learned the task significantly faster than nontreated controls (Fig. 1.4). In fact, the data suggest that animals that received combination therapy on a weekly basis beginning three months after ovariectomy performed as well as much younger ovariectomized controls, suggesting a complete prevention of age-related impairment on this task. In contrast, the same estradiol plus progesterone regimen was not as effective when initiated 10 months following ovariectomy. This suggests that the effects of estradiol on cognitive performance may diminish with age and time after ovarian function is lost.

Markowska and Savonenko (2002) have similarly reported that in middle-aged and aged rats, continuous estradiol treatment initiated nine months after ovariectomy did not significantly enhance working memory performance on a delayed nonmatching-to-position task, whereas continuous estradiol treatment did enhance performance when initiated eight months after ovariectomy and preceded for two months by repeated estradiol injections. Collectively, these data suggest that HT needs to be initiated within a set period of time (the "window of opportunity") to prevent age-related impairment of cognitive performance.

Based on these findings, Rapp et al. (2003) conducted a study in aged premenopausal monkeys to see if long-term cyclical estradiol treatment initiated after ovariectomy could prevent the effects of aging on specific measures of cognitive performance. Sixteen rhesus monkeys were ovariectomized at approximately 22 years of age. Half received a regimen of low-dose cyclical estradiol treatment and half received placebo. Over the course of treatment,

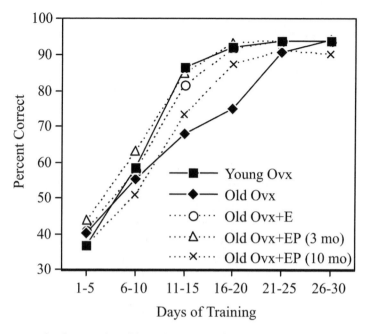

Fig. 1.4 Graphs showing that old rats (23–25 months of age) that were ovariectomized at 12 months of age and then placed immediately on continuous estradiol replacement (Ovx + E) or placed 3 months later on a continuing cyclic regimen of estradiol plus progesterone (Ovx + EP [3 mo]) acquired the DMP task as quickly as much younger (6 months old) ovariectomized controls. This same regimen of E + P was less effective when treatment was delayed and then initiated 10 months after ovariectomy (Ovx + EP [10 mo]). Values represent the mean percentage of correct responses for each group during each 5-day block of training.
Source: Adapted from Gibbs, 2000b, with permission from Elsevier.

animals were tested on a delayed response test of spatial working memory, a delayed nonmatching-to-sample recognition memory task, and an object discrimination learning task. The estradiol treatment substantially reversed a marked age-related impairment on the delayed response task and produced modest improvement on the delayed nonmatching-to-sample task. In contrast, estradiol treatment did not prevent age-related deficits in object discrimination learning, which were exacerbated by ovariectomy. These studies confirm and extend the rodent work showing that long-term estradiol treatment can help prevent age-related cognitive impairment, provided that treatment is initiated soon after loss of ovarian function.

Notably, a similar result was reported in humans. A three-year prospective observational study was conducted in Cache County, Utah (Zandi et al., 2002). A total of 1,866 women with a mean age of approximately 74.4 years were included in the analysis. Eight hundred of these women had never used HT. Of those who had used HT, most (72%) had used an unopposed oral estrogen preparation. Past estrogen use, but not current use, was associated with a significant reduction in the risk of developing AD (odds ratio = 0.33; 95% confidence interval: 0.15–0.65). In addition, the reduction in risk among past users increased with increasing duration of treatment, such that the apparent likelihood of developing AD was reduced 42 percent, 68 percent, and 83 percent among women who had used HT for less than 3 years, 3 to 10 years, and more than 10 years, respectively. These data support the conclusion that long-term HT therapy initiated around the time of menopause provides significant protection against age-related cognitive decline. The data also are consistent in suggesting that the effectiveness of HT declines with time following menopause. Hence, this study, along with the animal studies and a number of other human observational studies (reviewed in Sherwin, 2002), supports the idea that HT can significantly reduce the development of age-related dementia, provided that therapy is initiated at the appropriate time and in the appropriate regimen; however, the clinical evidence remains nondefinitive (Maki and Hogervorst, 2003; Mulnard et al., 2004).

Both the animal literature and the human literature are in agreement in suggesting that HT consisting of either estradiol or a combination of estradiol plus progestin can enhance performance within specific cognitive domains. Furthermore, evidence from both animal and human studies suggests that HT can reduce the incidence of age-related cognitive decline, provided that therapy is initiated within a specific period after the loss of ovarian function. The regimen of HT is also likely a critical factor, particularly with regard to combination estrogen plus progestin therapy. Precisely what the window of opportunity is in humans, and why sensitivity to estrogen therapy decreases with age and the long-term loss of ovarian function, still remain to be determined.

The Mechanisms of Estrogen's Effects on Cognitive Performance

Many different biological mechanisms have been proposed to contribute to estrogen-mediated effects on cognitive performance. Rather than provide a comprehensive review of all these potential mechanisms, this section focuses on two systems that have been the subject of considerable study, the hippocampal formation, and cholinergic projections from the basal forebrain.

Effects in the Hippocampus

The hippocampus is a medial temporal lobe structure that plays a critical role in memory consolidation, particularly declarative memory in humans, spatial working memory, and memories involving temporal contingencies in rodents (Zola-Morgan and Squire, 1993). The hippocampus receives indirect input from all sensory modalities and serves to integrate and reinforce specific patterns of neural activity within a widely distributed neocortical network, which forms the basis of long-term memories (Fries et al., 2003). One hippocampal cell type that has been extensively studied is the CA1 pyramidal cell, which is the primary output cell of the hippocampus.

CA1 pyramidal cells receive excitatory glutamatergic inputs from CA3 pyramidal cells, which form synaptic contacts with spines (primarily) located on CA1 cell apical dendrites. This is referred to as the Schaffer collateral-CA1 synapse. These synapses display several types of plasticity that are critical for hippocampal function and memory consolidation (Lynch, 2004). In addition, selective damage to CA1 pyramidal cells has been reported to produce a severe and selective learning deficit in humans (Zola-Morgan et al., 1986).

Estrogen has many effects on CA1 plasticity in rats. It increases excitability of the CA1 neurons (Rudick and Woolley, 2001; Wong and Moss, 1992), enhances long-term potentiation (LTP) and decreases long-term depression at the Schaffer collateral-CA1 synapse (Good et al., 1999; Vouimba et al., 2000; Warren et al., 1995), and leads to dramatic morphological changes in CA1 connections. Woolley and co-workers have shown that in young ovariectomized rats, two days of estrogen administration produces a significant increase (~30%) in the number of dendritic spines on the apical dendrites of CA1 pyramidal cells (reviewed in Woolley, 2000) (Fig. 1.5). The increased number of dendritic spines is associated with an increase in excitatory synaptic contacts with these cells, and specifically with an increase in new contacts as opposed to a strengthening of existing contacts (Yankova et al., 2001). This means that estrogen enhances the breadth of communication between CA1 pyramidal cells and divergent excitatory inputs. Estrogen also produces a substantial increase in N-methyl-D-aspartate (NMDA) receptor expression by CA1 pyramidal cells (Fig. 1.6), along with an increase in NMDA responses (Foy et al., 1999; Woolley et al., 1997). This increase is consistent with the fact

Control   **Estradiol**

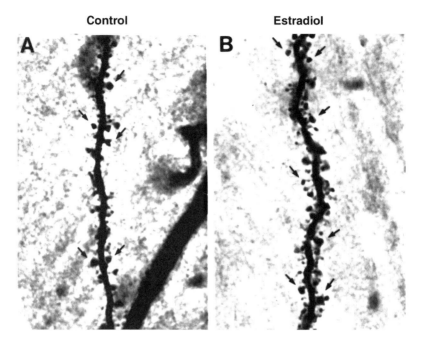

Fig. 1.5 Photomicrographs showing increased dendritic spine density on the dendrite of a CA1 pyramidal cell taken from an ovariectomized rat treated with estradiol (B) compared with an ovariectomized control (A). Dendritic segments are from the lateral branches of the apical dendritic tree of CA1 pyramidal cells. Some dendritic spines are indicated by arrows.
Source: Adapted from Woolley et al., 1997, © 1997 The Society for Neuroscience.

that the majority of the new synaptic contacts resulting from estrogen administration are glutamatergic and occur at NMDA receptor–containing sites. The NMDA receptor is critical to the occurrence of LTP at these sites (Morris et al., 1986). LTP is a form of synaptic plasticity characterized by a lasting potentiation of postsynaptic responses resulting from a burst of temporally associated excitatory input. Drugs that block LTP, either by acting at the NMDA receptors or by blocking downstream signal transduction mechanisms, significantly impair hippocampal effects on learning and memory (reviewed in Lynch, 2004). Estrogen has been shown to enhance LTP at the Schaffer collateral-CA1 synapse (Foy et al., 1999; Good et al., 1999), consistent with the increases in synaptic input and NMDA responses described.

Early studies showed that the effects of estradiol on CA1 plasticity are physiologically relevant and occur with a particular temporal sequence. For

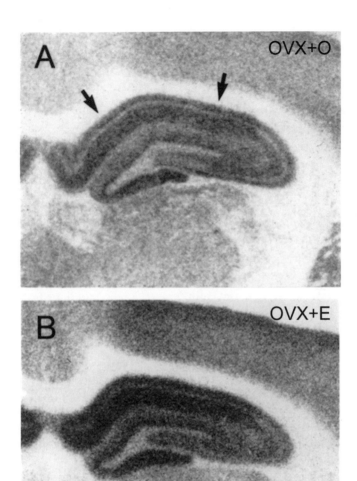

Fig. 1.6 Autoradiograms showing an increase in total [³H]glutamate binding in the hippocampus of ovariectomized rats treated with estradiol (B) compared with ovariectomized controls (A). Arrows indicate region CA1. Displacement with NMDA (not shown) reveals that the increase in glutamate binding produced by estradiol is attributable to enhanced NMDA binding.

Source: Adapted from Woolley et al., 1997, © 1997 The Society for Neuroscience.

example, in gonadally intact rats, the density of dendritic spines on the apical dendrites of the CA1 pyramidal cells decreases by approximately 30 percent between proestrus and estrus over the course of a five-day estrous cycle. This effect is mimicked by ovariectomy and can be prevented by the administration of estradiol (Gould et al., 1990). In ovariectomized rats, two days of estradiol treatment produces an increase in spine density on CA1 pyramidal neurons that peaks with approximately three days of estradiol treatment and then decays slowly to baseline over the next 10 to 14 days. Progesterone, when administered 24 hours after the last injection of estradiol, enhances the effect of estradiol on spine density within 2 hours of administration, but causes a rapid return to baseline levels within 24 hours, which would account for the rapid decline in spine density observed between proestrus and estrus (Woolley and McEwen, 1993). These findings demonstrate that the changes in connectivity produced by ovariectomy and estradiol and progesterone treatment are physiological as well as hormonally driven. Notably, similar effects of estradiol on spine density in CA1 pyramidal cells have been observed in young adult (but not old) rats (Adams et al., 2001) and in both young and old monkeys (Hao et al., 2003). Another study also reported an increase in spinophilin staining (a marker of dendritic spines) in layer I of area 46 prefrontal cortex in monkeys treated with estradiol, suggesting that the effects of estrogen on spine density are not restricted to area CA1 of the hippocampus (Tang et al., 2004). These results suggest that the effects on synaptic contacts may be relevant to the effects that loss of ovarian function and estradiol therapy have on brain aging and cognition in humans.

There also is evidence that the effects of estradiol and progesterone on spine density are relevant to effects on memory performance. Sandstrom and Williams (2001) evaluated the effects of estradiol and progesterone on short-term memory in ovariectomized rats using a modified Morris water maze task. Animals were tested for their ability to remember the location of a submerged platform 10, 30, and 100 minutes after training on successive days following hormone treatment. This design enabled the investigators to compare changes in short-term memory performance with the temporal changes in spine density previously reported. Studies showed that the animals' performance increased in response to estradiol and was greatest two to three days after administration (when CA1 spine density is at its peak), then decreased gradually toward baseline levels over the next five days. When progesterone was administered 24 hours after two consecutive days of estradiol treatment, performance again increased in response to estradiol, was greatest in animals tested several hours after progesterone administration (again, when CA1 spine density is at its peak), and returned to baseline levels 24 hours later. These results show a close temporal correlation between the effects of hormone treatment on spine density in CA1 and effects on memory performance.

Estrogen-Mediated Effects in the Hippocampus

Are the effects of estradiol on cognitive performance mediated by direct estrogen effects on hippocampal neurons? Several studies suggest that estradiol can act directly in the hippocampus to affect cognitive performance. In rats, intrahippocampal injections of estradiol administered immediately after training significantly enhanced memory performance on a Morris water maze task (Packard, 1998). Administration of estradiol two hours after training was not effective, suggesting that direct actions of estradiol in the hippocampus affected performance by enhancing memory consolidation, as opposed to affecting motivation or other performance parameters. Of note, an interaction with cholinergic afferents was also implicated. Dohanich et al. (G. P. Dohanich, personal communication, April 2004) recently showed that intrahippocampal administration of estradiol can also prevent deficits in radial arm maze performance produced by the systemic administration of scopolamine, again implicating an interaction between the effects of estradiol in the hippocampus and cholinergic afferents.

Both types of estrogen receptor (ER), ERα and ERβ, are expressed by hippocampal neurons (reviewed in McEwen, 2002). ERα is detected primarily in scattered γ-aminobutyric acid (GABA)–containing interneurons in the hippocampus, particularly in ventral hippocampus (Hart et al., 2001), and this distribution agrees nicely with the distribution of ER binding (Shughrue and Merchenthaler, 2000). ERβ mRNA has been detected primarily in pyramidal neurons (Shughrue et al., 1997) of Ammon's horn; however, only very weak ERβ immunoreactivity was detected in ventral CA2/3 (Shughrue and Merchenthaler, 2001).

Using primary neuronal cultures, Murphy and colleagues showed that the estrogen-mediated increase in dendritic spines involves the activation of phosphokinase A (PKA) and phosphorylation of cyclic AMP response element-binding protein (CREB) (Murphy and Segal, 1996, 1997). Selective inhibition of PKA or CREB phosphorylation completely prevented the estrogen-mediated increase in spines. Likewise, Lee et al. (2004) showed that estrogen stimulates phosphorylation of CREB in primary hippocampal cultures, that this effect is dependent on both MAPK and CaMK activities, and that estrogen-induced spinophilin expression in these cultures is blocked by KN93 (an inhibitor of CaMKII). These results are consistent with the observation that estrogen stimulates CREB phosphorylation via a number of pathways, including activation of MAPK (Wade and Dorsa, 2003) and CaMKII (Sawai et al., 2002). Some evidence suggests that CREB phosphorylation is also necessary for the maintenance of LTP (Deisseroth et al., 1996; Ying et al., 2002) and for memory consolidation (Guzowski and McGaugh, 1997).

Studies by Murphy and Segal (1996) showed that selective inhibition of NMDA receptors, but not AMPA/kainite receptors, prevents the estradiol-mediated increase in spines, which implicates Ca^{2+} entry via NMDA receptors as part of the mechanism by which estradiol stimulates spine formation. These effects may not be direct, as they are brought about by a significant reduction in GABA-mediated inhibition, associated with a substantial decrease (up to 80%) in the levels of glutamic acid decarboxylase within aspiny interneurons (Murphy et al., 1998). This suggests that disinhibition of the CA1 pyramidal neurons, via a reduction in GABA-mediated inhibitory signals, is an important early event in the estrogen-mediated increase in dendritic spines and synapses on CA1 pyramidal cells.

Rudick and Woolley (2001) confirmed that the administration of estradiol (10 μg of estradiol given subcutaneously) produces significant disinhibition of CA1 pyramidal cells within 24 hours through a reduction in the amplitude and frequency of $GABA_A$ receptor–mediated inhibitory currents. Specifically, using hippocampal slice cultures prepared from estradiol- and vehicle-treated rats, Rudick et al. showed that estradiol produced a reduction in the amplitude of evoked inhibitory postsynaptic currents (IPSCs) and a reduction in the frequency of spontaneous miniature IPSCs. These effects were completely dependent on tamoxifen-sensitive estrogen receptors (Rudick et al., 2003), consistent with the presence of ERα within GABAergic interneurons located in the hippocampus. The effects were also transient: by 72 hours, inhibition was restored to control levels, by which time spine density and NMDA responses are enhanced. Cholinergic afferents were likewise implicated in the estrogen-mediated disinhibition of CA1 pyramidal neurons, again implicating cholinergic afferents in the effects of estradiol on hippocampal function.

Collectively, these studies provide strong evidence that estrogen-mediated effects on cognitive performance, particularly tasks that rely on hippocampal-mediated memory consolidation, are due at least in part to estrogen effects on hippocampal connectivity and excitability. The data support a model in which estrogen-mediated effects on the structure and function of CA1 pyramidal cells result from transient disinhibition of the cells brought about by a reduction in GABA-mediated inhibitory currents, resulting in increased excitability of CA1 pyramidal cells, activation of MAPK and CaMKII, and phosphorylation of CREB.

Estrogen and Basal Forebrain Cholinergic Neurons

In addition to the effects of estrogen on hippocampal connectivity and function, there is increasing evidence that cholinergic projections play an important role in estrogen-mediated effects on cognitive performance. Cholinergic neurons in the medial septum (MS) and nucleus basalis magnocellularis (NBM) are the primary source of cholinergic innervation to the hippocampus and cerebral cortex (Mesulam, 1996). These neurons are well documented to play an important role in learning, memory, and attentional processes (Baxter and Chiba, 1999; Everitt and Robbins, 1997). Selective lesions of corticopetal cholinergic projections from the NBM to the cerebral cortex have been shown to impair performance on specific measures of social memory, such as social transmission of food preferences (Berger-Sweeney et al., 2000; Vale-Martinez et al., 2002), acquisition of a negative patterning task (Butt et al., 2000), recognition of offspring by olfaction in sheep (Ferreira et al., 2001), and learning of simple visual discriminations in monkeys (Ridley et al., 1999a). Cholinergic projections from the NBM have also been shown to play a role in inhibitory avoidance learning, both via projections to the amygdala and via projections to the cerebral cortex (reviewed in Power et al., 2003), and have been shown to be heavily involved in attentional processes, as revealed by tasks that measure vigilance and selective attention (reviewed in Sarter et al., 2003).

Cholinergic projections to the hippocampus also play an important role in cognitive processes, although the specific processes that are affected are somewhat less clear. Studies have shown significant impairment in the acquisition of specific spatial tasks and working memory performance following selective injections of 192IgG-saporin into the MS (Shen et al., 1996; Walsh et al., 1996); however, many studies disagree and have shown little effect of confined septal cholinergic lesions on working memory performance (Baxter and Chiba, 1999). We recently showed that in rats, loss of cholinergic neurons in the MS impairs acquisition of a delayed matching-to-position T-maze task (Johnson et al., 2002), with a magnitude of effect similar to impairments observed in aged animals. In monkeys, selective destruction of cholinergic input to the hippocampus impairs learning of visuospatial conditional discriminations, but not simple visual discriminations (Ridley et al., 1999a). Notably, combined lesions of cholinergic neurons in the MS and NBM produced more robust cognitive impairments in both rats and monkeys than were observed after destruction of one or the other cholinergic system, implying some redundancy among the cholinergic projection systems (Pizzo et al., 2002; Ridley et al., 1999b; Wrenn et al., 1999). Both the septohippocampal and the corticopetal projections are impaired in association with aging and AD, and this impairment is thought to contribute significantly to the etiology of age-related cognitive decline (Linstow and Platt, 1999; Smith et al., 1999).

Ovariectomy has a negative impact on basal forebrain cholinergic neurons in rats, as demonstrated by decreases in choline acetyltransferase (ChAT) activity, high-affinity choline uptake, and acetylcholine release (Gibbs, 2000c). In addition, long-term loss of ovarian function produces decreases in trkA and ChAT mRNA in MS and NBM beyond the effects of normal aging (Gibbs, 1998). TrkA is a tyrosine kinase receptor that specifically binds nerve growth factor, a target-derived trophic factor that supports the survival and function of basal forebrain cholinergic neurons. TrkA expression decreases significantly with age and loss of ovarian function in rats (Gibbs, 1998, 2003), and is significantly reduced in persons with AD (Mufson et al., 1997). In addition, short-term knockdown of trkA protein reduces the expression of specific cholinergic markers and produces an impairment in contextual fear conditioning (Woolf et al., 2001). These data suggest that decreased trkA expression could be a major factor contributing to cholinergic impairment and age-related cognitive decline. We hypothesize that by exacerbating the decrease in trkA, loss of estradiol accelerates age-related impairment in cholinergic function, thereby contributing to age-related cognitive decline.

Studies also have shown that estradiol treatment can increase the functionality of basal forebrain cholinergic projections in rats, as demonstrated by increases in ChAT mRNA and protein, high-affinity choline uptake, and potassium-stimulated acetylcholine release (Gabor et al., 2003; Gibbs, 2001). Recent studies in nonhuman primates have likewise shown significant increases in ChAT immunostaining within select basal forebrain cholinergic neurons in both young and aged ovariectomized monkeys receiving short-term estrogen treatment (Kompoliti et al., 2004). Studies in rats show that the effects of estradiol on acetylcholine release are lasting with long-term continuous treatment (Table 1.1), and may be the best indicator of sustained estrogen-mediated effects on cholinergic function. Notably, estradiol consistently af-

TABLE 1.1

Effects of Estradiol on Basal and Potassium-Stimulated Acetylcholine Release in the Hippocampus of Ovariectomized Rats

Session 1		Session 2	
No E (n = 4)		E (n = 4)	
Basal ACh release	0.56 ± 0.15	Basal ACh release	0.64 ± 0.28
Increase with high potassium	75.0 ± 27.6%	Increase with high potassium	212.4 ± 50.4%*
E (n = 6)		No E (n = 6)	
Basal ACh release	0.34 ± 0.14	Basal ACh release	0.52 ± 0.16
Increase with high potassium	192.0 ± 43.5%*	Increase with high potassium	94.2 ± 32.8%

Source: Adapted from Gabor et al., 2003, with permission from Elsevier.

Note: Ovariectomized rats received Silastic capsules containing 17β-estradiol or sham surgery. In vivo microdialysis was conducted after six to seven weeks of treatment to measure basal and potassium-stimulated acetylcholine (ACh) release in the hippocampus. Animals then underwent a second procedure during which all E-treated animals had their estrogen capsules removed and all non-E-treated animals received Silastic capsules containing 17β-estradiol. Six weeks later, in vivo microdialysis was repeated. Values for basal release represent pmol ACh/20 μL of dialysate. Treatment with estradiol resulted in significantly greater potassium-stimulated ACh release regardless of treatment order and estradiol had no significant effect on basal release.
*$p < 0.05$ relative to non-E-treated animals.

fects stimulated release, but not basal release, suggesting that the administration of estradiol enhances the release of acetylcholine during periods of demand without affecting basal cholinergic tone.

Studies in rats also suggest that the effects of estradiol on the cholinergic neurons are dose dependent, with low physiological doses being the most effective (Gibbs, 1997), and that effects vary as a function of the specific regimen of hormone treatment. For example, one study evaluated the effects of different regimens of treatment on high-affinity choline uptake in the hippocampus and frontal cortex of young adult, ovariectomized rats (Gibbs, 2000a). The regimens most effective at increasing levels of high-affinity choline uptake were cyclical administration of estradiol plus progesterone and continuous administration of estradiol alone (Fig. 1.7). The least effective regimen was the continuous, simultaneous administration of estradiol plus progesterone, which had a small though nonsignificant negative effect on high-affinity choline uptake. Collectively, these studies demonstrate that estradiol and progesterone can have a positive effect on basal forebrain cholinergic function, provided that an appropriate dose and regimen are used.

Precisely how estradiol affects basal forebrain cholinergic neurons is still not known. The effects could be either direct or indirect. In rats, estrogen receptors (primarily ERα) have been detected in a subset of the cholinergic neurons (Miettinen et al., 2002; Shughrue et al., 2000), although specific ER-mediated regulation of gene expression within these neurons has not been

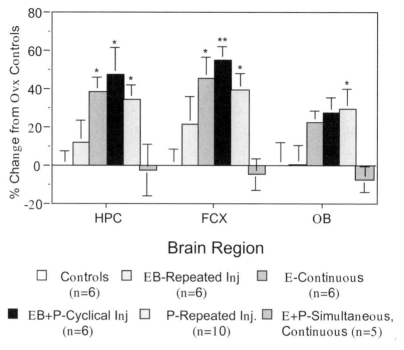

Brain Region

☐ Controls   ☐ EB-Repeated Inj   ☐ E-Continuous
   (n=6)   (n=6)   (n=6)

■ EB+P-Cyclical Inj   ☐ P-Repeated Inj.   ☐ E+P-Simultaneous,
   (n=6)   (n=10)   Continuous (n=5)

Fig. 1.7 Effects of different regimens of hormone replacement therapy on high-affinity choline uptake in different regions of the rat brain. Rats were ovariectomized and treated with hormones or vehicle for 2 weeks. Values represent the mean percentage change relative to controls ± SEM. Note that continuous estradiol administration and repeated administration of estradiol plus progesterone were most effective, whereas continuous simultaneous treatment with estradiol plus progesterone was least effective. HPC, hippocampus; FCX, frontal cortex; OB, olfactory bulbs. $^{*}P < 0.05$, $^{**}P < 0.01$ relative to controls.
Source: Gibbs and Gabor, 2003. Reprinted with permission.

reported. Recently, Pongrac et al. (2004) evaluated the effects of estradiol on cholinergic markers using primary neuronal cultures of embryonic basal forebrain. In these cultures, treatment with estradiol produced a dose-related increase in high-affinity choline uptake and acetylcholine production, in the absence of any effect on ChAT. The increase in high-affinity choline uptake was blocked by ICI182780 (an inhibitor of both ERα and ERβ), was associated with an increase in phosphoERK1/2, and was blocked by U0126, an inhibitor of MEK. These data suggest that estradiol can enhance acetylcholine production by increasing high-affinity choline uptake via a mechanism involving ER-mediated activation of the MAP kinase signaling pathway.

Similarly, Dominguez et al. (2004) showed that estradiol increases the length and branching of cholinergic fibers in embryonic basal forebrain cultures, and that this effect is associated with an increase in phosphoERK1/2 and is blocked by U0126. Hence, estradiol may also affect cholinergic fiber outgrowth via a mechanism involving ER-mediated activation of the MAP kinase signaling pathway. Whether estradiol has the same effect on cholinergic neurons in the adult brain is still unknown. In monkeys, these same neurons reportedly do not express immunoreactivity for ERα (Blurton-Jones et al., 1999; Mufson et al., 1999), even though estradiol increases ChAT staining within the rostral cholinergic cell group (Kompoliti et al., 2004). In this case, the cholinergic neurons might be affected indirectly by changes in growth factor production, the expression of growth factor receptors, or changes in the activity of GABAergic or serotonergic afferents. Although there is some evidence to support each of these possibilities, definitive evidence that one particular mechanism accounts for the effects of estradiol on basal forebrain cholinergic function has not yet been reported.

Evidence That Effects on Cholinergic Neurons Are Functionally Relevant

Although it is not known precisely how estradiol affects basal forebrain cholinergic neurons, many studies provide compelling evidence that the effects of estradiol on cholinergic function are directly relevant to effects on cognitive performance. For example, in rats, estradiol has been shown to reduce impairments on T-maze and radial arm maze tasks produced by either systemic or intrahippocampal administration of scopolamine, a muscarinic receptor blocker (Fader et al., 1999; Gibbs, 1999). Studies by Packard (1998) show that the memory-enhancing effect produced by injecting estradiol directly into the hippocampus is blocked by systemic administration of scopolamine and enhanced by systemic administration of oxotremorine (a muscarinic receptor agonist), demonstrating cholinergic modulation of estrogen effects in the hippocampus. Studies by Marriott and Korol (2003) show that estradiol increases acetylcholine release in the hippocampus during place learning. As with stimulated release, estradiol affected release only while animals were performing the task, and did not affect basal cholinergic tone. In rats, selective destruction of the cholinergic neurons projecting to the hippocampus not only produced a learning impairment but also prevented the estradiol-mediated enhancement of learning on a delayed matching-to-position

T-maze task (Gibbs, 2002), demonstrating that cholinergic projections to the hippocampus are necessary for estradiol to enhance learning on this task.

In monkeys, studies have shown small but significant changes in the density of cholinergic afferents within specific regions of the prefrontal cortex in response to ovariectomy and estradiol treatment. In particular, studies show that cholinergic fiber density decreases within layer II of prefrontal cortex following ovariectomy and is fully restored following either short-term (Kritzer and Kohama, 1999) or long-term (two years) (Tinkler et al., 2004) estradiol treatment. Notably, long-term (two years) ovariectomy and estradiol treatment did not affect cholinergic fiber density in parietal cortex. These findings may account for the observation that in monkeys, estradiol restored normal sensitivity to scopolamine on a visuospatial attention task, but did not alter the effect of scopolamine on a delayed response task (Voytko, 2000, 2002; Voytko and Tinkler, 2004).

Collectively, these findings suggest that cholinergic projections from the basal forebrain play a very important role in estradiol-mediated effects on cognitive performance. What, then, is the relationship between the effects of estrogen on cholinergic function and on the hippocampus?

Cholinergic Afferents and Effects of Estradiol on Hippocampal Function

Perhaps the most exciting recent development in this field has been the discovery that the effects of estradiol on basal forebrain cholinergic neurons and on hippocampal function are related (i.e., that basal forebrain cholinergic afferents play an important role with respect to estradiol-mediated effects on the structure and function of hippocampal circuits). For example, Rudick et al. (2003) demonstrated that the estradiol-mediated disinhibition of CA1 pyramidal cells is greatly reduced by selective destruction of cholinergic neurons in MS. This means that the ability of estradiol to reduce GABAergic inhibition of CA1 pyramidal cells depends to a large degree on the presence and functionality of these cholinergic neurons. Given that disinhibition of the CA1 pyramidal cells is thought to underlie the estradiol-mediated increase in synaptic density and excitability of these cells, one would predict that the loss of cholinergic afferents would likewise prevent the estradiol-mediated changes in hippocampal connectivity and function.

Confirmative studies by Leranth and co-workers have shown that elimination of the cholinergic afferents, either by fimbria/fornix transection (Leranth et al., 2000) or by immunotoxic lesion of the cholinergic neurons (Lam and Leranth, 2003), completely prevents the estradiol-mediated increase in spine density on CA1 pyramidal cells, without affecting spine density in non-estrogen-treated animals. Likewise, Daniel and Dohanich (2001) showed that administration of an M2 muscarinic receptor antagonist completely blocked the estradiol-mediated increase in NMDA binding in CA1, as well as the estradiol-mediated enhancement of working memory performance on a radial arm maze task. Conversely, enhancement of cholinergic activity with physostigmine increased NMDA binding in CA1 to the same degree as estradiol administration.

These results support a model in which estrogen-mediated enhancement of cholinergic activity originating in the basal forebrain enables structural and functional changes to occur in the hippocampus and cortex, changes that underlie specific estrogen-mediated effects on cognitive performance. This model is consistent with emerging evidence that cholinergic afferents play a critical role in enabling structural plasticity to occur in somatosensory (Prakash et al., 2004), auditory (Weinberger, 2003), and visual cortices (Bear and Singer, 1986). The model is also consistent with data showing that the effects of estradiol on CA1 dendritic spines are diminished in aged rats (Adams et al., 2001), which reportedly have impaired cholinergic function. Hence, according to this model, the ability of estrogen to enhance basal forebrain cholinergic function is fundamental to its ability to enhance cognitive performance, and perhaps to prevent or delay the development of age-related cognitive decline.

The Effects of Progesterone

To this point, the discussion has focused on the effects of estradiol. Much less is known about the effects of progestins, or the interaction between estrogens and progestins, on cognitive performance. Progestins can be sedating, and typically have a negative effect on affect and mood. Our own studies, however, showed that long-term cyclical administration of estradiol and progesterone prevented age-related cognitive decline in young adult rats tested on a delayed matching-to-position T-maze task as effectively as continuous estradiol treatment (Gibbs, 2000b). Similarly, Markham and Juraska (2002) showed that simultaneous administration of estradiol and progesterone was as effective as estradiol alone at reducing forgetting on a reference memory version of a Morris water maze task in middle-aged ovariectomized rats. In contrast, Chesler and Juraska (2000) showed that acute sequential administration of estradiol followed by progesterone had a significant negative impact on the same reference memory version of the Morris water maze task in young adult rats, even though there was no effect of estradiol or progesterone alone. In addition, Warren and Juraska (2000) reported that aged rats in constant estrus performed better on a spatial version of the Morris water maze task than aged pseudopregnant rats, suggesting that progesterone inhibits spatial learning in aged animals. Hence, the effects of progesterone on cognitive performance in young and aged rats are not straightforward. It is likely that specific cognitive effects depend on the effects on cortical circuits, and on the role of those circuits in the specific tasks being assessed.

For example, in the hippocampus, progesterone initially enhances the effects of estradiol on dendritic spine density in area CA1, but then reduces spine density to control levels within 24 hours after progesterone administration (Woolley and McEwen, 1993). Consistent with these effects, Sandstrom and Williams (2001) showed that performance on a modified Morris water maze task was first enhanced after progesterone administration and then declined.

Our own studies have shown that progesterone can have positive effects on basal forebrain cholinergic neurons and that repeated cyclical administration of progesterone enhances the effects of estradiol on basal forebrain cholinergic function (Gibbs, 2000a), consistent with effects observed on the delayed matching-to-position T-maze task. In contrast, adding continuous progesterone administration simultaneously with continuous estradiol appears to have a negative effect on basal forebrain cholinergic neurons (Gibbs, 2000a), which we predict would have a negative impact on spatial learning. This result suggests that the regimen of treatment, in addition to the task, may be critical in determining the net effect of combination therapy on cognitive function (see chapter 2).

The choice of progestin may also be critical in determining effects on brain function and cognitive performance. Medroxyprogesterone acetate is a synthetic α-hydroxyprogesterone analog that is routinely prescribed in combination with CEE. MPA binds with high affinity to the progesterone receptor, but it also has glucocorticoid and androgenic effects (Bamberger et al., 1999; Bentel et al., 1999; Hackenberg et al., 1993; Selman et al., 1996). Both the administration of glucocorticoid (Hu et al., 1996; Wahba and Soliman, 1992) and acute stress (Wahba and Soliman, 1992) have been shown to decrease ChAT activity in the basal forebrain, which may contribute to negative effects on the performance of specific tasks.

In one study, Rice et al. (2000) compared the effects of CEE and CEE plus MPA on cognitive performance in a group of older postmenopausal Japanese-

American women. Over a two-year period, women receiving CEE performed better on tests of global cognitive performance, abstract reasoning, and category fluency than controls. In contrast, women receiving CEE plus MPA performed significantly worse on measures of global cognitive performance and mental tracking than controls. This result suggests that over a two-year period, MPA prevented specific positive effects of estrogen and had a negative impact on cognitive performance. Whether these effects are related to negative effects on basal forebrain cholinergic function is unknown; however, the findings are consistent with reported effects on basal forebrain cholinergic neurons, and may be directly relevant to the effects of combination therapy on the risk for dementia detected in the WHIMS trial (Shumaker et al., 2003).

The point of this discussion is that progesterone has been reported to have both positive and negative effects on cognitive performance, as well as specific effects on cortical circuits implicated in effects on learning and memory. In addition, the effects of any given progestin on cognitive performance are likely to depend not only on the specific tasks being assessed but also on the choice of progestin and the regimen (cyclical versus continuous) of treatment. While in vitro studies are beginning to identify in more detail the effects of different progestins on neuronal processes in culture (see chapter 5), much more study of the effects of progestins on neural circuits is needed in order to develop a better understanding of the potential effects on cognitive performance.

Relevance to the WHIMS Data

Given the very strong animal data showing positive effects of HT on cognitive performance and the prevention of age-related cognitive decline, how do we account for the WHIMS data showing that women who received HT consisting of CEE and MPA were twice as likely to develop probable dementia over a five-year period as women who received placebo (Shumaker et al., 2003)? The answer, we believe, resides in what the animal literature tells us about the effects of HT on neural systems involved in cognitive performance.

First, there is the evidence that the ability of estrogen to enhance cognitive performance diminishes with age and time after the loss of ovarian function, and that there is a window of opportunity during which HT must be initiated in order to be effective. Precisely what this window of opportunity is in humans is not known; however, all of the women included in the WHIMS trial were 65 years old or older, and hence an average of 10 to 12 years postmenopause. We suggest that age 65 years is beyond the window of opportunity for HT to produce beneficial effects on cognitive performance and that administration of HT to women whose age places them beyond the window of opportunity explains the failure to reliably detect the variety of positive effects typically seen in animal studies. This formulation is supported by the results of the Cache County study discussed earlier (Zandi et al., 2002) and by the many other observational studies that have detected significant reductions in the risk of Alzheimer-related dementia among women who have received postmenopausal HT (reviewed in Sherwin, 2002), although studies increasingly show that HT in older women does not appear to be effective (Mulnard et al., 2004).

Second, there is the evidence that basal forebrain cholinergic neurons play an important role in estrogen-mediated effects on cognitive performance, and that the effects of estrogen on basal forebrain cholinergic neurons vary as a function of the dose and regimen of HT. Ovariectomized rats treated either continuously with estradiol or cyclically with estradiol and progesterone showed the greatest increase in high-affinity choline uptake, whereas animals treated continuously and simultaneously with estradiol and progesterone displayed a small decrease in high-affinity choline uptake. It should be noted that continuous and simultaneous treatment with both estradiol and progesterone most closely resembles the treatment regimen used in the combination-therapy arm of the WHIMS trial.

We recently evaluated the effects of long-term treatment with CEE and CEE plus MPA on levels of ChAT and acetylcholinesterase in the MS of cynomolgus monkeys (Gibbs et al., 2002). As noted earlier, MPA is a synthetic progestin that, in addition to binding to the progesterone receptor, has both glucocorticoid and androgenic effects. Monkeys were ovariectomized and received either CEE (Premarin) or CEE plus MPA once daily in their food for two years. Doses were calculated based on caloric intake to approximate a dose of 0.625 mg of CEE and 2.5 mg of MPA used in women, and closely approximated the combined estrogen plus progesterone regimen used in the WHIMS trial. The levels of ChAT and acetylcholinesterase were significantly reduced in the MS of animals treated with CEE plus MPA (Fig. 1.8), suggesting that long-term daily administration of CEE plus MPA has a negative impact on cholinergic neurons in the basal forebrain. In contrast, levels were not significantly affected by treatment with CEE alone.

Based on these results, we predict that long-term combination therapy of the type used in the WHIMS trial would have a negative impact on age-related cognitive decline. This is precisely what has been reported. Therefore, rather

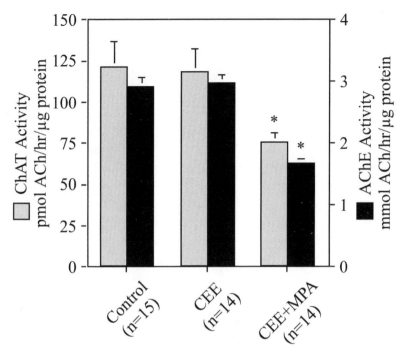

Fig. 1.8 Effects of long-term treatment with conjugated equine estrogens (CEE) or CEE plus medroxyprogesterone acetate (MPA) on choline acetyltransferase (ChAT) and acetylcholinesterase (AChE) activities in the medial septum of ovariectomized cynomolgus monkeys. Values represent group mean ± SEM. Note that long-term daily administration of E + P resulted in significant reductions in the levels of both ChAT and AChE. *$P < 0.05$ relative to ovariectomized controls.
Source: Gibbs and Gabor, 2003. Reprinted with permission.

than contradicting the animal studies, the WHIMS data, along with the many recent observational studies, help to confirm the validity of the animal studies, which collectively support the benefits of HT with respect to brain aging and cognition, provided that therapy is initiated at the appropriate time, and at a dose and in a regimen appropriate for the brain. This analysis does not explain all of the results of the WHIMS trial, however. For example, the WHIMS trial also showed that women treated with CEE alone had a greater risk for dementia and global cognitive decline, particularly women with lower cognitive ratings at the start of treatment (Espeland et al., 2004; Shumaker et al., 2004). Why CEE alone would have a negative effect on cognition in postmenopausal women is not clear, although the effect may be secondary to adverse cardiovascular effects. Clearly, further study of the mechanisms that underlie hormonal effects on cognitive performance is needed.

Based on our analysis, we conclude that the WHIMS data, particularly the data for the combined CEE plus MPA arm of the study, are consistent with the results of recent animal studies, and we propose that the negative effects of combination therapy can be explained by a number of factors, including the age of the women at the time the study was initiated, the regimen of CEE plus MPA administered, and the use of MPA as the progestin.

Conclusions

Animal studies provide compelling evidence that, after the loss of ovarian function, HT consisting of either estradiol or a combination of estradiol plus progesterone can enhance cognitive performance and reduce age-related cognitive decline. Several plausible biological mechanisms for these effects have been identified. At present, there is compelling evidence that estrogen-mediated disinhibition of hippocampal CA1 pyramidal cells results in structural and functional changes in hippocampal circuits and that these changes underlie at least some of the effects on spatial learning, short-term working memory, and memory consolidation that have been described. Furthermore, studies show that these effects depend on cholinergic afferents from the basal forebrain, which also are affected significantly by ovariectomy and estradiol treatment. These data support a model in which estrogen-mediated enhancement of cholinergic activity originating in the basal forebrain enables structural and functional changes to occur in the hippocampus and cortex, which changes underlie specific estrogen-mediated effects on cognitive performance. In addition, there is compelling evidence for the effects of ovariectomy and estrogen therapy on both serotonergic and dopaminergic systems in the brain, particularly with respect to serotonergic neurons in the dorsal raphe and monoaminergic innervation of the prefrontal cortex. It is likely that these effects also contribute to the effects of HT on mood and cognition. Consequently, the animal data suggest that HT should have a beneficial effect on brain function and cognition in postmenopausal women.

The animal studies also suggest that HT must be initiated within a limited period after the loss of ovarian function in order to be effective. Most prospective trials that have focused on prevention, including the WHIMS trial, have focused exclusively on effects in women age 65 years or older, which we believe is past the window of opportunity for eliciting a beneficial effect of HT on cognitive performance. In addition, animal studies suggest that the regimen of HT is extremely important and that, in contrast to the beneficial effects of estradiol alone or cyclical administration of estradiol and progesterone, long-term simultaneous combination therapy is not beneficial and may have adverse effects on basal forebrain cholinergic function and cognition. These findings are consistent with many of the recent observational studies conducted in humans and help to account for the negative effect of CEE plus MPA on dementia observed in the recent WHIMS trial. Despite these negative findings, we predict that postmenopausal HT can help to prevent age-related cognitive decline in women, provided that therapy is initiated around the time of menopause, at a dose and in a regimen appropriate for the brain.

REFERENCES

Adams MM, Shah RA, Janssen WG, et al. 2001. Different modes of hippocampal plasticity in response to estrogen in young and aged female rats. Proc Natl Acad Sci USA 98:8071–76.
Balschun D, Wolfer DP, Gass P, et al. 2003. Does cAMP response element-binding protein have a pivotal role in hippocampal synaptic plasticity and hippocampus-dependent memory? J Neurosci 23:6304–14.
Bamberger CM, Else T, Bamberger AM, et al. 1999. Dissociative glucocorticoid activity of medroxyprogesterone acetate in normal human lymphocytes. J Clin Endocrinol Metab 84:4055–61.
Baxter MG, Chiba AA. 1999. Cognitive functions of the basal forebrain. Curr Opin Neurobiol 9:178–83.
Bear MF, Singer W. 1986. Modulation of visual cortical plasticity by acetylcholine and noradrenaline. Nature 320:172–76.
Bentel JM, Birrell SN, Pickering MA, et al. 1999. Androgen receptor agonist activity of the synthetic progestin, medroxyprogesterone acetate, in human breast cancer cells. Mol Cell Endocrinol 154:11–20.
Berger-Sweeney J, Stearns NA, Frick KM, et al. 2000. Cholinergic basal forebrain is critical for social transmission of food preferences. Hippocampus 10:729–38.
Bimonte HA, Denenberg VH. 1999. Estradiol facilitates performance as working memory load increases. Psychoneuroendocrinology 24:161–73.
Birke LI. 1979. Object investigation by the oestrous rat and guinea-pig: the oestrous cycle and the effects of oestrogen and progesterone. Anim Behav 27(Pt 2):350–58.
Blurton-Jones MM, Roberts JA, Tuszynski MH. 1999. Estrogen receptor immunoreactivity in the adult primate brain: neuronal distribution and association with p75, trkA, and choline acetyltransferase. J Comp Neurol 405:529–42.

Brookmeyer R, Gray S, Kawas C. 1998. Projections of Alzheimer's disease in the United States and the public health impact of delaying disease onset. Am J Public Health 88:1337–42.

Butt AE, Allen K, Arthur K, et al. 2000. A test of negative patterning reveals selective impairment in configural association learning in rats with 192 IgG-saporin lesions of the nucleus basalis magnocellularis (abstr). Soc Neurosci 26:563.5.

Chesler EJ, Juraska JM. 2000. Acute administration of estrogen and progesterone impairs the acquisition of the spatial Morris water maze in ovariectomized rats. Horm Behav 38:234–42.

Daniel JM, Dohanich GP. 2001. Acetylcholine mediates the estrogen-induced increase in NMDA receptor binding in CA1 of the hippocampus and the associated improvement in working memory. J Neurosci 21:6949–56.

Daniel JM, Roberts SL, Dohanich GP. 1999. Effects of ovarian hormones and environment on radial maze and water maze performance of female rats. Physiol Behav 66:11–20.

Deisseroth K, Bito H, Tsien RW. 1996. Signaling from synapse to nucleus: postsynaptic CREB phosphorylation during multiple forms of hippocampal synaptic plasticity. Neuron 16:89–101.

Dohanich GP. 2002. Gonadal steroids, learning and memory. In *Hormones, Brain and Behavior,* ed. DW Pfaff, AP Arnold, AM Etgen, et al., 1:265–327. San Diego: Academic Press.

Dominguez R, Jalali C, de Lacalle S. 2004. Morphological effects of estrogen on cholinergic neurons in vitro involves activation of extracellular signal-regulated kinases. J Neurosci 24:982–90.

Espeland MA, Rapp SR, Shumaker SA, et al. 2004. Conjugated equine estrogens and global cognitive function in postmenopausal women: Women's Health Initiative Memory Study. JAMA 291:2959–68.

Everitt BJ, Robbins TW. 1997. Central cholinergic systems and cognition. Annu Rev Psychol 48:649–84.

Fader AJ, Johnson PEM, Dohanich GP. 1999. Estrogen improves working but not reference memory and prevents amnestic effects of scopolamine on a radial-arm maze. Pharmacol Biochem Behav 62:711–17.

Farquhar CM, Steiner CA. 2002. Hysterectomy rates in the United States, 1990–1997. Obstet Gynecol 99:229–34.

Ferreira G, Meurisse M, Gervais R, et al. 2001. Extensive immunolesions of basal forebrain cholinergic system impair offspring recognition in sheep. Neuroscience 106:103–15.

Foy MR, Xu J, Xie X, et al. 1999. 17beta-estradiol enhances NMDA receptor-mediated EPSPs and long-term potentiation. J Neurophysiol 81:925–29.

Frick KM, Fernandez SM, Bulinski SC. 2002. Estrogen replacement improves spatial reference memory and increases hippocampal synaptophysin in aged female mice. Neuroscience 115:547–58.

Fries P, Fernandez G, Jensen O. 2003. When neurons form memories. Trends Neurosci 26:123–24.

Gabor R, Nagle R, Johnson DA, et al. 2003. Estrogen enhances potassium-stimulated acetylcholine release in the rat hippocampus. Brain Res 962:244–47.

Gibbs RB. 1997. Effects of estrogen on basal forebrain cholinergic neurons vary as a function of dose and duration of treatment. Brain Res 757:10–16.

Gibbs RB. 1998. Impairment of basal forebrain cholinergic neurons associated with aging and long-term loss of ovarian function. Exp Neurol 151:289–302.

Gibbs RB. 1999. Estrogen replacement enhances acquisition of a spatial memory task and reduces deficits associated with hippocampal muscarinic receptor inhibition. Horm Behav 36:222–33.

Gibbs RB. 2000a. Effects of gonadal hormone replacement on measures of basal forebrain cholinergic function. Neuroscience 101:931–38.

Gibbs RB. 2000b. Long-term treatment with estrogen and progesterone enhances acquisition of a spatial memory task by ovariectomized aged rats. Neurobiol Aging 21:107–16.

Gibbs RB. 2000c. Oestrogen and the cholinergic hypothesis: implications for oestrogen replacement therapy in postmenopausal women. In *Neuronal and Cognitive Effects of Oestrogens*, ed. J Goode. Novartis Found Symp 230:94–111.

Gibbs RB. 2001. Potential mechanisms for the effects of estrogen on cognitive processes: Role of basal forebrain cholinergic projections. In *Neuroplasticity, Development, and Steroid Hormone Action*, ed. RJ Handa, S Hayashi, E Teresawa, et al., 117–29. Boca Raton: CRC Press.

Gibbs RB. 2002. Basal forebrain cholinergic neurons are necessary for estrogen to enhance acquisition of a delayed matching-to-position t-maze task. Horm Behav 42: 245–57.

Gibbs RB. 2003. Effects of aging, ovariectomy, and long-term hormone replacement on cholinergic neurons in the medial septum and nucleus basalis magnocellularis. J Neuroendocrinol 15:477–85.

Gibbs RB, Gabor R. 2003. Estrogen and cognition: applying preclinical findings to clinical perspectives. J Neurosci Res 74:637–43.

Gibbs RB, Nelson D, Anthony MS, et al. 2002. Effects of long-term hormone replacement and of tibolone on choline acetyltransferase and acetylcholinesterase activities in the brains of ovariectomized, cynomologus monkeys. Neuroscience 113:907–14.

Good M, Day M, Muir JL. 1999. Cyclical changes in endogenous levels of oestrogen modulate the induction of LTD and LTP in the hippocampal CA1 region. Eur J Neurosci 11:4476–80.

Gould E, Woolley CS, Frankfurt M, et al. 1990. Gonadal steroids regulate dendritic spine density in hippocampal pyramidal cells in adulthood. Neuroscience 10:1286–91.

Granholm AC, Ford KA, Hyde LA, et al. 2002. Estrogen restores cognition and cholinergic phenotype in an animal model of Down syndrome. Physiol Behav 77:371–85.

Guzowski JF, McGaugh JL. 1997. Antisense oligodeoxynucleotide-mediated disruption of hippocampal cAMP response element binding protein levels impairs consolidation of memory for water maze training. Proc Natl Acad Sci USA 94:2693–98.

Hackenberg R, Hawighorst T, Filmer A, et al. 1993. Medroxyprogesterone acetate inhibits the proliferation of estrogen- and progesterone-receptor negative MFM-223 human mammary cancer cells via the androgen receptor. Breast Cancer Res Treat 25:217–24.

Hao J, Janssen WG, Tang Y, et al. 2003. Estrogen increases the number of spinophilin-immunoreactive spines in the hippocampus of young and aged female rhesus monkeys. J Comp Neurol 465:540–50.

Hart SA, Patton JD, Woolley CS. 2001. Quantitative analysis of ER alpha and GAD colocalization in the hippocampus of the adult female rat. J Comp Neurol 440:144–55.

Heikkinen T, Puolivali J, Liu L, et al. 2002. Effects of ovariectomy and estrogen treatment on learning and hippocampal neurotransmitters in mice. Horm Behav 41:22–32.

Henderson VW. 2000. Oestrogens and dementia. In *Neuronal and Cognitive Effects of Oestrogens,* ed. J Goode. Novartis Found Symp 230:254–73.

Hendrie HC. 1998. Epidemiology of dementia and Alzheimer's disease. Am J Geriatr Psychiatry 6(2 Suppl 1):S3–S18.

Hogervorst E, De Jager C, Budge M, et al. 2004. Serum levels of estradiol and testosterone and performance in different cognitive domains in healthy elderly men and women. Psychoneuroendocrinology 29:405–21.

Hogervorst E, Williams J, Budge M, et al. 2000. The nature of the effect of female gonadal hormone replacement therapy on cognitive function in post-menopausal women: a meta-analysis. Neuroscience 101:485–512.

Hogervorst E, Yaffe K, Richards M, et al. 2002. Hormone replacement therapy for cognitive function in postmenopausal women. Cochrane Database Syst Rev 3:CD003122.

Hu ZT, Yuri K, Ichikawa T, et al. 1996. Exposure of postnatal rats to glucocorticoids suppresses the development of choline acetyltransferase-immunoreactive neurons: role of adrenal steroids in the development of forebrain cholinergic neurons. J Chem Neuroanat 10:1–10.

Johnson DA, Zambon NZ, Gibbs RB. 2002. Selective lesion of cholinergic neurons in the medial septum by 192 IgG-saporin impairs learning in a delayed matching to position T-maze paradigm. Brain Res 943:132–41.

Kompoliti K, Chu Y, Polish A, et al. 2004. Effects of estrogen replacement therapy on cholinergic basal forebrain neurons and cortical cholinergic innervation in young and aged ovariectomized rhesus monkeys. J Comp Neurol 472:193–207.

Kritzer MF, Kohama SG. 1999. Ovarian hormones differentially influence immunoreactivity for dopamine beta-hydroxylase, choline acetyltransferase, and serotonin in the dorsolateral prefrontal cortex of adult rhesus monkeys. J Comp Neurol 409:438–51.

Lam TT, Leranth C. 2003. Role of the medial septum diagonal band of Broca cholinergic neurons in oestrogen-induced spine synapse formation on hippocampal CA1 pyramidal cells of female rats. Eur J Neurosci 17:1997–2005.

LeBlanc ES, Janowsky J, Chan BK, et al. 2001. Hormone replacement therapy and cognition: systematic review and meta-analysis. JAMA 285:1489–99.

Lee SJ, Campomanes CR, Sikat PT, et al. 2004. Estrogen induces phosphorylation of cyclic AMP response element binding (pCREB) in primary hippocampal cells in a time-dependent manner. Neuroscience 124:549–60.

Leranth C, Shanabrough M, Horvath TL. 2000. Hormonal regulation of hippocampal spine synapse density involves subcortical mediation. Neuroscience 101:349–56.

Li C, Brake WG, Romeo RD, et al. 2004. Estrogen alters hippocampal dendritic spine shape and enhances synaptic protein immunoreactivity and spatial memory in female mice. Proc Natl Acad Sci USA 101:2185–90.

Linstow EV, Platt B. 1999. Biochemical dysfunction and memory loss: the case of Alzheimer's dementia. Cell Mol Life Sci 55:601–16.

Luine VN, Jacome LF, Maclusky NJ. 2003. Rapid enhancement of visual and place memory by estrogens in rats. Endocrinology 144:2836–44.

Lynch MA. 2004. Long-term potentiation and memory. Physiol Rev 84:87–136.

Maki P, Hogervorst E. 2003. The menopause and HRT: HRT and cognitive decline. Best Pract Res Clin Endocrinol Metab 17:105–22.

Marin R, Guerra B, Hernandez-Jimenez JG, et al. 2003. Estradiol prevents amyloid-beta peptide-induced cell death in a cholinergic cell line via modulation of a classical estrogen receptor. Neuroscience 121:917–26.

Markham JA, Juraska JM. 2002. Aging and sex influence the anatomy of the rat anterior cingulate cortex. Neurobiol Aging 23:579–88.

Markham JA, Pych JC, Juraska JM. 2002. Ovarian hormone replacement to aged ovariectomized female rats benefits acquisition of the Morris water maze. Horm Behav 42:284–93.

Markowska AL, Savonenko AV. 2002. Effectiveness of estrogen replacement in restoration of cognitive function after long-term estrogen withdrawal in aging rats. J Neurosci 22:10985–95.

Marriott LK, Korol DL. 2003. Short-term estrogen treatment in ovariectomized rats augments hippocampal acetylcholine release during place learning. Neurobiol Learn Mem 80:315–22.

McEwen B. 2002. Estrogen actions throughout the brain. Recent Prog Horm Res 57: 357–84.

Mesulam MM. 1996. The systems-level organization of cholinergic innervation in the human cerebral cortex and its alterations in Alzheimer's disease. Prog Brain Res 109:285–97.

Miettinen RA, Kalesnykas G, Koivisto EH. 2002. Estimation of the total number of cholinergic neurons containing estrogen receptor-alpha in the rat basal forebrain. J Histochem Cytochem 50:891–902.

Morris RG, Anderson E, Lynch GS, et al. 1986. Selective impairment of learning and blockade of long-term potentiation by an N-methyl-D-aspartate receptor antagonist, AP5. Nature 319:774–76.

Mufson EJ, Cai WJ, Jaffar S, et al. 1999. Estrogen receptor immunoreactivity within subregions of the rat forebrain: neuronal distribution and association with perikarya containing choline acetyltransferase. Brain Res 849:253–74.

Mufson EJ, Lavine N, Jaffar S, et al. 1997. Reduction in p140-TrkA receptor protein within the nucleus basalis and cortex in Alzheimer's disease. Exp Neurol 146: 91–103.

Mulnard RA, Corrada MM, Kawas CH. 2004. Estrogen replacement therapy, Alzheimer's disease, and mild cognitive impairment. Curr Neurol Neurosci Rep 4:368–73.

Murphy DD, Cole NB, Greenberger V, et al. 1998. Estradiol increases dendritic spine density by reducing GABA neurotransmission in hippocampal neurons. J Neurosci 18:2550–59.

Murphy DD, Segal M. 1996. Regulation of dendritic spine density in cultured rat hippocampal neurons by steroid hormones. J Neurosci 16:4059–68.

Murphy DD, Segal M. 1997. Morphological plasticity of dendritic spines in central neurons is mediated by activation of cAMP response element binding protein. Proc Natl Acad Sci USA 94:1482–87.

Packard MG. 1998. Posttraining estrogen and memory modulation. Horm Behav 34: 126–39.

Pizzo DP, Thal LJ, Winkler J. 2002. Mnemonic deficits in animals depend upon the degree of cholinergic deficit and task complexity. Exp Neurol 177:292–305.

Pongrac JL, Gibbs RB, Defranco DB. 2004. Estrogen-mediated regulation of cholinergic expression in basal forebrain neurons requires extracellular-signal-regulated kinase activity. Neuroscience 124:809–16.

Power AE, Vazdarjanova A, McGaugh JL. 2003. Muscarinic cholinergic influences in memory consolidation. Neurobiol Learn Mem 80:178–93.

Prakash N, Cohen-Cory S, Penschuck S, et al. 2004. Basal forebrain cholinergic system is involved in rapid nerve growth factor (ngf)-induced plasticity in the barrel cortex of adult rats. J Neurophysiol 91:424–37.

Rapp PR, Morrison JH, Roberts JA. 2003. Cyclic estrogen replacement improves cognitive function in aged ovariectomized rhesus monkeys. J Neurosci 23:5708–14.

Rice MM, Graves AB, McCurry SM, et al. 2000. Postmenopausal estrogen and estrogen-progestin use and 2-year rate of cognitive change in a cohort of older Japanese American women: the Kame Project. Arch Intern Med 160:1641–49.

Ridley RM, Barefoot HC, Maclean CJ, et al. 1999a. Different effects on learning ability after injection of the cholinergic immunotoxin ME20.4IgG-saporin into the diagonal band of Broca, basal nucleus of Meynert, or both in monkeys. Behav Neurosci 113: 303–15.

Ridley RM, Pugh P, Maclean CJ, et al. 1999b. Severe learning impairment caused by combined immunotoxic lesion of the cholinergic projections to the cortex and hippocampus in monkeys. Brain Res 836:120–38.

Rudick CN, Gibbs RB, Woolley CS. 2003. A role for the basal forebrain cholinergic system in estrogen-induced disinhibition of hippocampal pyramidal cells. J Neurosci 23:4479–90.

Rudick CN, Woolley CS. 2001. Estrogen regulates functional inhibition of hippocampal CA1 pyramidal cells in the adult female rat. J Neurosci 21:6532–43.

Sandstrom NJ, Williams CL. 2001. Memory retention is modulated by acute estradiol and progesterone replacement. Behav Neurosci 115:384–93.

Sarter M, Bruno JP, Givens B. 2003. Attentional functions of cortical cholinergic inputs: what does it mean for learning and memory? Neurobiol Learn Mem 80:245–56.

Sawai T, Bernier F, Fukushima T, et al. 2002. Estrogen induces a rapid increase of calcium-calmodulin-dependent protein kinase II activity in the hippocampus. Brain Res 950:308–11.

Selman PJ, Wolfswinkel J, Mol JA. 1996. Binding specificity of medroxyprogesterone acetate and proligestone for the progesterone and glucocorticoid receptor in the dog. Steroids 61:133–37.

Shen J, Barnes CA, Wenk GL, et al. 1996. Differential effects of selective immunotoxic lesions of medial septal cholinergic cells on spatial working and reference memory. Behav Neurosci 110:1181–86.

Sherwin BB. 2002. Estrogen and cognitive aging in women. Trends Pharmacol Sci 23:527–34.

Shughrue PJ, Merchenthaler I. 2000. Evidence for novel estrogen binding sites in the rat hippocampus. Neuroscience 99:605–12.

Shughrue PJ, Merchenthaler I. 2001. Distribution of estrogen receptor beta immunoreactivity in the rat central nervous system. J Comp Neurol 436:64–81.

Shughrue P, Scrimo P, Lane M, et al. 1997. The distribution of estrogen receptor-beta mRNA in forebrain regions of the estrogen receptor-alpha knockout mouse. Endocrinology 138:5649–52.

Shughrue PJ, Scrimo PJ, Merchenthaler I. 2000. Estrogen binding and estrogen receptor characterization (ERα and ERβ) in the cholinergic neurons of the rat basal forebrain. Neuroscience 96:41–49.

Shumaker SA, Legault C, Kuller L, et al. 2004. Conjugated equine estrogens and incidence of probable dementia and mild cognitive impairment in postmenopausal women: Women's Health Initiative Memory Study. JAMA 291:2947–58.

Shumaker SA, Legault C, Rapp SR, et al. 2003. Estrogen plus progestin and the incidence of dementia and mild cognitive impairment in postmenopausal women: the Women's Health Initiative Memory Study: a randomized controlled trial. JAMA 289: 2651–62.

Smith DE, Roberts J, Gage FH, et al. 1999. Age-associated neuronal atrophy occurs in the primate brain and is reversible by growth factor gene therapy. Proc Natl Acad Sci USA 96:10893–98.

Tang Y, Janssen WG, Hao J, et al. 2004. Estrogen replacement increases spinophilin-immunoreactive spine number in the prefrontal cortex of female rhesus monkeys. Cereb Cortex 14:215–23.

Tinkler GP, Tobin JR, Voytko ML. 2004 Effects of two years of estrogen loss or replacement on nucleus basalis cholinergic neurons and cholinergic fibers to the dorsolateral prefrontal and inferior parietal cortex of monkeys. J Comp Neurol 469: 507–21.

Vale-Martinez A, Baxter MG, Eichenbaum H. 2002. Selective lesions of basal forebrain cholinergic neurons produce anterograde and retrograde deficits in a social transmission of food preference task in rats. Eur J Neurosci 16:983–98.

Vouimba RM, Foy MR, Foy JG, et al. 2000. 17beta-estradiol suppresses expression of long-term depression in aged rats. Brain Res Bull 53:783–87.

Voytko ML. 2000. The effects of long-term ovariectomy and estrogen replacement therapy on learning and memory in monkeys (*Macaca fascicularis*). Behav Neurosci 114:1078–87.

Voytko ML. 2002. Estrogen and the cholinergic system modulate visuospatial attention in monkeys (*Macaca fascicularis*). Behav Neurosci 116:187–97.

Voytko ML, Tinkler GP. 2004. Cognitive function and its neural mechanisms in non-human primate models of aging, Alzheimer disease, and menopause. Front Biosci 9:1899–914.

Wade CB, Dorsa DM. 2003. Estrogen activation of cyclic adenosine 5'-monophosphate response element-mediated transcription requires the extracellularly regulated kinase/mitogen-activated protein kinase pathway. Endocrinology 144:832–38.

Wahba ZZ, Soliman KFA. 1992. Effect of stress on choline-acetyltransferase activity of the brain and the adrenal of the rat. Experientia 48(3):65–68.

Walsh TJ, Herzog CD, Gandhi C, et al. 1996. Injection of IgG 192-saporin into the medial septum produces cholinergic hypofunction and dose-dependent working memory deficits. Brain Res 726:69–79.

Warren SG, Humphreys AG, Juraska JM, et al. 1995. LTP varies across the estrous cycle: enhanced synaptic plasticity in proestrus rats. Brain Res 703:26–30.

Warren SG, Juraska JM. 2000. Sex differences and estropausal phase effects on water maze performance in aged rats. Neurobiol Learn Mem 74:229–40.

Weinberger NM. 2003. The nucleus basalis and memory codes: auditory cortical plasticity and the induction of specific, associative behavioral memory. Neurobiol Learn Mem 80:268–84.

Wilson IA, Puolivali J, Heikkinen T, et al. 1999. Estrogen and NMDA receptor antagonism: effects upon reference and working memory. Eur J Pharmacol 381(2–3):93–99.

Wong M, Moss RL. 1992. Long-term and short-term electrophysiological effects of estrogen on the synaptic properties of hippocampal CA1 neurons. J Neurosci 12:3217–25.

Woolf NJ, Milov AM, Schweitzer ES, et al. 2001. Elevation of nerve growth factor and antisense knockdown of TrkA receptor during contextual memory consolidation. J Neurosci 21:1047–55.

Woolley CS. 2000. Effects of oestradiol on hippocampal circuitry. Novartis Found Symp 230:173–80 [discussion 181–87].

Woolley CS, McEwen BS. 1993. Roles of estradiol and progesterone in regulation of hippocampal dendritic spine density during the estrous cycle in the rat. J Comp Neurol 336:293–306.

Woolley CS, Weiland NG, McEwen BS, et al. 1997. Estradiol increases the sensitivity of hippocampal CA1 pyramidal cells to NMDA receptor-mediated synaptic input: correlation with dendritic spine density. J Neurosci 17:1848–59.

Wrenn CC, Lappi DA, Wiley RG. 1999. Threshold relationship between lesion extent of the cholinergic basal forebrain in the rat and working memory impairment in the radial maze. Brain Res 847:284–98.

Xu H, Gouras GK, Greenfield JP, et al. 1998. Estrogen reduces neuronal generation of Alzheimer beta-amyloid peptides. Nat Med 4:447–51.

Yankova M, Hart SA, Woolley CS. 2001. Estrogen increases synaptic connectivity be-tween single presynaptic inputs and multiple postsynaptic CA1 pyramidal cells: a serial electron-microscopic study. Proc Natl Acad Sci USA 98:3525–30.

Ying SW, Futter M, Rosenblum K, et al. 2002. Brain-derived neurotrophic factor induces long-term potentiation in intact adult hippocampus: requirement for ERK activa-tion coupled to CREB and upregulation of Arc synthesis. J Neurosci 22:1532–40.

Zandi PP, Carlson MC, Plassman BL, et al. 2002. Hormone replacement therapy and incidence of Alzheimer disease in older women: the Cache County Study. JAMA 288:2123–29.

Zola-Morgan S, Squire LR. 1993. Neuroanatomy of memory. Annu Rev Neurosci 16: 547–63.

Zola-Morgan S, Squire LR, Amaral DG. 1986. Human amnesia and the medial temporal region: enduring memory impairment following a bilateral lesion limited to field CA1 of the hippocampus. J Neurosci 6:2950–67.

CHAPTER TWO

The Short-Lived Effects of Hormone Therapy on Cognitive Function

EVA HOGERVORST, Ph.D.

Dementia is characterized by severe memory and other cognitive deficits that interfere with daily life. Alzheimer disease (AD), the most prevalent type of dementia, is characterized by a slow and progressive decline (McKhann et al., 1984). Abundant evidence from in vitro and in vivo animal studies suggests that estrogens could act favorably on almost all mechanisms known to be affected in cognitive decline and AD (see chapter 1; for a review, see Henderson, 2004). The biological plausibility that estrogen therapy (ET) could protect the aging brain in postmenopausal women has been called its strongest suit (Barrett-Connor, 1998). Possibly no other substance has held such promise in the treatment or prevention of AD. The initial enthusiasm for ET's potential was further fueled by observational studies indicating that women taking hormone therapy (HT) were at lower risk for dementia and had better cognitive function than were nonusers (Hogervorst et al., 2000; LeBlanc et al., 2001; Yaffe, Sawaya, et al., 1998). The results of the largest treatment study to date to investigate this possibility, the Women's Health Initiative Memory Study (WHIMS), however, have induced many women to discontinue HT. In that study, ET was found to increase the risk for dementia, stroke, and breast cancer. This chapter focuses on what remains of the original hypothesis that ET or HT could have positive effects on cognitive function in postmenopausal women.

Observational Studies
Risk Reduction for AD with the Use of HT

Many cross-sectional studies have shown that women without dementia are twice as likely to use HT as women with AD. Prospective cohort studies indicate that HT users also have half the risk of developing AD as nonusers (Hogervorst et al., 2000). The discrepancy between the outcome of large, multicenter, well-designed, randomized, placebo-controlled trials (RCTs) and observational studies could indicate potential confounds in either. We will first discuss some of the most important potential sources of bias in the observational studies, which may have confounded the association between HT use and AD, and then analyze potential confounds of the treatment studies in more detail.

Confounds for Observational Studies of AD Cases:
Recall and Prescription Bias

Odds ratios are assessed by comparing the percentages of HT users and nonusers in cases (here, patients with AD) and controls. The use of HT can be assessed subjectively by asking participants or their families about current or past use. It can also be assessed objectively by checking medical pharmaceutical records or other documentary proof of use (such as prescription labels, which can be checked by asking women to bring their prescriptions to the laboratory) or by assessing serum estrogen levels.

Because of the nature of the disease, women with dementia might be less able to recall their HT use, which could confound the association reported. In our meta-analyses (Hogervorst et al., 2000), studies in which information on HT use was obtained from family members or surrogate responders overall reported a lower use of HT in patients than studies that used other means of acquiring data on HT use. We tested whether the protective effect of HT in 14 observational studies related to the method of assessing HT use. The odds ratio (OR) was less in the six studies that used patient responses (OR = 0.43, 95% confidence interval [CI]: 0.32–0.57, heterogeneity test: χ^2 (5) = 7.55, P = 0.18) compared to those studies that used surrogate responders (OR = 0.66, 95% CI: 0.48–0.91, heterogeneity test: χ^2 (5) = 11.94, P = 0.04) or computerized medical files (OR = 0.78, 95% CI: 0.51–1.19, heterogeneity test: χ^2 (1) = 5.12, P = 0.02). In addition, one recent study using medical pharmaceutical prescription records at baseline with a follow-up of 3,924 participants found that 20 percent of women with AD or cognitive impairment who had also been classified as HT users by prescription did not recall their HT use, compared with 9 percent of controls (Petitti et al., 2002). This finding indicates that women with AD systematically underestimate their own HT use. Finally, once women have acquired AD, physicians may be more reluctant to prescribe HT, in the expectation of poor adherence to the treatment regimen out of forgetfulness.

Confounds for Observational Studies of AD Cases: Publication Bias

Although mostly protective effects of HT were reported in studies published between 1994 and 1999 (Balderischi et al., 1998; Henderson et al., 1994; Kawas et al., 1996; Lerner et al., 1997; Mortel and Meyer, 1995; Paganini-Hill and Henderson, 1994; Slooter et al., 1999; Tang et al., 1996; Waring et al., 1999), in recent years several large observational studies did not find overall positive effects of HT (Petitti et al., 2002; Seshadri et al., 2001; Zandi et al., 2002), similar to studies done before 1995 (Amaducci et al., 1986; Borenstein-Graves et al., 1990; Brenner et al., 1994; Broe et al., 1990; Heyman et al., 1984). This pattern could suggest that a tendency to publish mainly positive results may have been a confounding factor in the mid- to late 1990s.

Cognitive Function and Cognitive Decline in Women

Many cross-sectional and prospective cohort studies have reported positive associations between HT use and cognitive function in women without dementia (Hogervorst et al., 2000). These results, however, are subject to potential sources of bias that are also applicable to studies investigating the association between HT and the incidence and prevalence of AD. These potentially confounding factors include the healthy-user bias, level of educational achievement, and socioeconomic status (SES).

Confounds for Observational Studies of Cognitive Function
and Decline: Healthy-User Bias

Observational cross-sectional studies of women without dementia and prospective studies relating the incidence of AD to HT may have been confounded in ways that are hard to control statistically. For example, women could decide to take HT as part of a healthy lifestyle, which in itself could protect against AD and cognitive decline. An eight-year prospective study that initially enrolled premenopausal women found that those women who decided to use HT at menopause were more highly educated and already had lower blood pressure, cholesterol levels, and plasma insulin levels, weighed less, consumed less alcohol, and exercised more before menopause set in than women who never used HT (Matthews et al., 1996). A Danish prospective study also reported that future HT users had better cognitive performance before treatment was initiated than never users (Lokkegaard et al., 2002).

Confounds for Observational Studies of Cognitive Function and Decline: SES and Education

Many observational studies are biased because they included mainly white, highly educated women (e.g., the Baltimore Longitudinal Study of Aging, the Cache County Study, the Leisure World cohort). HT users in general have higher levels of education and SES than women who do not use HT (Barrett-Connor, 1998). This could protect them against cognitive decline and AD because of healthier lifestyles associated with a high level of education and SES (i.e., they would be expected to have more knowledge about healthy food and to have financial access to better foods and supplements, medical care, exercise opportunities, and leisure time).

Surprisingly, an earlier review (Hogervorst et al., 2000) found that cohort studies of women without dementia that included women with a lower SES and less education (Jacobs et al., 1998) reported greater advantages for HT users than for nonusers, even when these factors were controlled for. However, the inclusion of women of lower SES, most of whom would not have used HT, could have artificially created a larger difference. This effect may be particularly salient in the United States, where prescription drugs often have to be paid for by the individual because of insurance restrictions or lack of coverage. One of the problems may be that HT statistically acted as an "umbrella variable" that could explain all the variance of the other factors, because it is so closely linked to the combination of education, SES, and related healthy lifestyle factors.

Socioeconomic status is an independent (but highly related) factor of the educational influences on aging (Barrett-Connor, 1998). In our review, 17 of the 18 observational studies we examined had controlled for education. The only study that did not find an effect of HT on cognition, however, was also the only study that did not control for education (Paganini-Hill and Henderson, 1996). This result could indicate that the effects of HT are stronger in women with less education. This interaction was reported in another study (Matthews et al., 1999). Women with less education may have fewer resources to cope with cognitive decline and may therefore be more at risk for AD. ET could potentially enhance residual physiological resources (through its effect on cholinergic function, nerve growth factors, and dendritic outgrowth) and would be particularly useful in this vulnerable group. Post hoc analyses of existing treatment studies might indicate whether this is the case. Analyses stratified for education in the WHIMS study, however, did not indicate that treatment would have been beneficial for women with low levels of education (Shumaker et al., 2003).

In sum, several important confounds, such as lower recall of HT use, prescription bias, publication bias, and a generally less healthy lifestyle associated with not using HT, could have been responsible for the observational findings that suggest that HT is associated with a lower risk for AD and better cognitive function in women without dementia.

Observational Studies of Estrogen Levels, Cognitive Function, and Women with AD

The original rationale for giving women ET after menopause to prevent cognitive decline was the belief that estrogen deficiency was a risk factor for AD. Several studies reported low levels of estradiol (E_2, the most potent estrogen) in women with AD compared with controls (Fillit et al., 1986; Manly et al., 2000). This finding was not replicated in the well-characterized Oxford Project to Investigate Memory and Ageing (OPTIMA) cohort. In fact, total E_2 levels were slightly higher in women with AD (Hogervorst et al., 2003).

That high levels of estrogen may not necessarily protect the aging brain is reflected in the fact that elderly age-matched men have much higher levels of E_2 and testosterone (which can be converted into E_2 in the brain) than postmenopausal women (Hogervorst, De Jager, et al., 2004). Several observational studies have shown that elderly men experience a steeper decline in cognitive function and have lower cognitive performance than women. This is particularly true for verbal memory functions (Barrett-Connor and Kritz-Silverstein, 1999; Cerhan et al., 1998; Hogervorst, Bandelow, et al., 2004). Verbal memory was hypothesized to be most sensitive to estrogen effects (Sherwin, 1994).

On the other hand, one could argue that women have about twice the risk of developing AD as men (Launer et al., 1999) because of their lower levels of sex hormones. In our study of 150 elderly men and women without dementia, positive associations were found between endogenous estradiol levels and performance on verbal memory tasks in women but not in men. This result is in line with the results of some studies (Drake et al., 2000; Wolf and Kirschbaum, 2002) and could suggest that estrogen protects women (but not men) without dementia against cognitive decline. However, others did not find a positive association between estrogen levels and verbal memory in women without dementia (Barrett-Connor and Goodman-Gruen, 1999; Carlson and Sherwin, 1998; Polo-Kantola et al., 1998). Our review of observational studies that investigated the association between endogenous hormone levels and cognitive function in elderly women without dementia found no consistent evidence that low levels of endogenous estrogens related to poor cognitive performance (Hogervorst et al., 2000). However, it was concluded that higher bioavailable (unbound) E_2 levels could be a better variable than total E_2 to predict slower cognitive change over time (Yaffe, Lui, et al., 2000).

Treatment Studies
The Treatment of Women with AD

By the mid-1990s, when optimism over the benefits of ET was at its height, several small treatment studies all seemed to suggest that HT could improve cognitive functions of women with and without dementia. Most of these studies had methodological problems, however, and were of relatively short duration (Hogervorst et al., 2000; Yaffe, Sawaya, et al., 1998). By the end of the 1990s, the tide seemed to be turning. In 2000, three RCTs with a total of 212 women with AD (Henderson et al., 2000; Mulnard et al., 2000; Wang et al., 2000) showed that HT did not improve their cognitive abilities or prevent their cognitive decline. Although our meta-analyses showed an initial improvement after two to three months of treatment, after one year some of the measures seemed to indicate an accelerated cognitive decline in the women with AD who had been taking HT (Hogervorst et al., 2002b).

The Treatment of Women without Dementia: The WHIMS Study

The largest RCT to date, the Women's Health Initiative Memory Study, showed a doubled risk for dementia in women who had been randomized to HT (Shumaker et al., 2003). Women using HT also did not show the improvement in cognitive function over time that the placebo users had shown (Rapp et al., 2003). The WHIMS study included more than 4,000 women age 65 years and older. These women did not have dementia at baseline and were followed up for four years on average. The results of this study suggest that prescribing HT could result in an additional 23 cases of dementia per 10,000 women per year (Shumaker et al., 2003). Because the risk for ischemic stroke was also

1.5 times higher in women who had been randomized to HT, it was suggested that silent infarcts may have mediated the increased risk for dementia (Shumaker et al., 2003). Risk factors for cerebrovascular disease are often the same as those for AD and cognitive decline, and when cerebrovascular disease is present, less AD pathology is needed to induce cognitive deficits (Hogervorst et al., 2002). Earlier results of the WHI study had led to discontinuation of the estrogen plus progestagen arm, for it was found that in women taking HT, the risk of an adverse coronary heart disease event increased by 29 percent and the risk of stroke increased by 41 percent. There was also an increased risk of breast cancer, with an additional eight more women in the treatment group having developed invasive breast cancer compared to placebo users (Rymer et al., 2003). These results of the WHI study also led to the abrupt cessation of the Women's International Study of Long Duration Estrogen after Menopause (WISDOM; Wren, 1998), a similar study conducted in the United Kingdom. The risks were increased most after the first year after enrollment, however, which could suggest that randomization had not been optimal, with more women having been randomized to the treatment group who were in the preliminary stages of dementia. The type of screening instrument used in WHIMS does not have adequate specificity to detect these early cases, particularly if the women have high levels of educational achievement (Hogervorst et al., 2000).

In February 2004, the estrogen-only arm of the WHI study was discontinued, and preliminary results were published in April (Anderson et al., 2004). Although the risk for breast cancer was not increased in women using estrogen only, there was a similar trend toward an increased risk for dementia, and there was still an increased risk for stroke, with an absolute excess risk of 12 additional strokes per 10,000 person-years. Differences between groups were highest after the first year (OR = 3.06 and OR = 1.37 at year 2) but had reversed direction after three years (OR = 0.67). Risks again increased after four and five years (OR = 1.70, OR = 1.84) and were in the reverse direction after six years (OR = 0.96). Thus, risks were not consistent over time, and in both studies, CEE alone and CEE plus medroxyprogesterone acetate (MPA), there were no additional cases with mild cognitive impairment in the treatment group. Because many of these individuals are thought to be in the preliminary stages of AD, this group would have been expected to have increased significantly if HT increased the risk for dementia. Although these issues may be important, to date the WHI study is the largest controlled study, and it did not show the positive effects expected of HT.

In integrating the WHIMS findings with existing research and trying to explain the recent negative findings in the light of the earlier positive ones, we will focus on two main questions: Could other treatment regimens have led to a different outcome? Or could particular characteristics of the women treated have led to a different outcome? In the next section we address these questions using our updated quantitative conservative meta-analyses (Hogervorst et al., 2002a, 2002b) and qualitative analyses, which included studies that could not be added to the meta-analyses. With these additional data at hand, we consider the following possible explanations for the negative WHIMS results:

1a. After the WHIMS results were published, several investigators suggested that the treatment regimen was responsible for the negative effects. For instance, the addition of a progestagen could have been responsible for reversing positive estrogenic effects.

1b. Others suggested it was the type of estrogen used in WHIMS (i.e., Premarin or conjugated synthetic estrogens) or mode of administration (oral versus bolus or transdermal) that was not effective.

2a. Women enrolled in the WHIMS study may have been too old to benefit from treatment. Animal studies (see chapter 1) suggest that there is a window of time (immediately after the onset of menopause) when treatment is effective.

2b. Alternatively, there may be subgroups of women (e.g., relatively young, surgically menopausal women) in whom treatment would be indicated.

2c. It is possible that the treatment effects are modified by other variables, such as genetic or lifestyle variables. Possibly treatment could be useful for women who are genetically at risk for AD. Perhaps lifelong exposure to estrogens is more important than relatively short-duration estrogen treatment after the onset of menopause.

Some alternatives to HT in the treatment of cognitive deficiency are discussed at the end of this chapter.

Explaining the Negative Outcome of WHIMS
Treatment Regimens

As chapter 1 indicates, different treatment regimens may have different effects on the brain. The following sections discuss the type of estrogen and progesterone used and the timing and mode of administration of treatment.

The Addition of a Progesterone

Premarin (or conjugated equine estrogens, or CEE) was the treatment used in the WHI study, in WISDOM, and in several other large RCTs (e.g., PREPARE). The main reason for using Premarin was pragmatic: most women in the United States were prescribed this drug for menopausal complaints. It was also argued that because the observational studies showed decreased risks for AD, most of those women would have also used Premarin. MPA is added to CEE in a standard treatment package for women with an intact uterus to prevent endometrial cancer; however, MPA may not have been a good choice, in light of its known negative effects on cardiovascular disease (Sarrel, 1989). This association could explain the increased risk of stroke and infarcts in WHIMS. The most recent data from WHIMS suggest that MPA may have been responsible, because the risk for stroke was smaller and the risk for coronary heart disease (CHD) was not increased in women who had received CEE only (Anderson et al., 2004).

Similarly, an earlier RCT, the Heart and Estrogen/Progestin Replacement Study (HERS, n = 2,763) found that of women who had CHD and who were followed up for an average of four years, those who had been randomly assigned to CEE plus MPA had worse performance on tests of verbal fluency than those assigned to the placebo arm. No differences were seen on tests of global cognitive function, speed of information processing, or verbal memory (Grady et al., 2002). Two earlier, smaller RCTs (Binder et al., 2001; Goebel et al., 1995) of CEE and MPA versus placebo did not find any positive or negative effects on cognitive function after eight and nine months in the respective studies.

A limited number of observational studies reported that the addition of a progestagen to ET was not necessarily associated with negative effects on cognitive function (Hogervorst et al., 2000). It is possible that the type of progestagen used is related to less favorable effects and that a different progestagen would have made a difference in WHIMS. The results of animal studies (see chapter 1) underline this theory. Apart from potential vascular effects, MPA can also decrease cholinergic function, which may be one of the more important effects of estrogens on the aging brain. Studies suggesting that extended continuous treatment with MPA plus CEE might thus have prevented the positive effects of estrogen were reviewed in chapter 1.

Positive effects on cognitive function have been reported in three studies in which an estradiol (E_2) was used in combination with a progestagen other than MPA. In a small study reported by Linzmayer et al. (2001), 49 postmenopausal women between the ages of 46 and 67 years who had insomnia related to menopause were given placebo, oral E_2 valerate alone, or oral E_2 valerate in combination with a relatively new progestin, Dienogest, for two months. The authors noted, "estradiol, and even more in combination with Dienogest, improved verbal and visual memory, which is in line with the improvement in information processing speed and capacity objectified by event-related potentials." The differences, however, were small, and significance could not be replicated in our conservative Cochrane meta-analyses (Hogervorst et al., 2002a). Two other studies conducted in relatively young, symptomatic, postmenopausal women who were treated with oral E_2 and norgestrel (Fedor-Freyberg, 1977) or oral E_2 and progestagen (Hogervorst et al., 1999) reported positive effects on verbal memory and other cognitive functions. These results accord with the observational studies that did not find that the addition of a progestagen resulted in negative results (Hogervorst et al., 2000).

In sum, several studies using an E_2 with a progestagen other than MPA found positive effects on cognitive function. Apart from the addition of MPA, the difference in outcome could thus depend on the type of estrogen used.

Different Estrogen Treatments

Meta-analyses carried out before the results of the WHIMS study were reported had already shown that CEE, with or without MPA, never had a positive effect on cognition in women without dementia (Hogervorst et al., 2002b) and led to only short-term improvement of two to three months in women with dementia (Hogervorst et al., 2002a). Longer-term studies of women with dementia indicated that the positive effects of CEE on some measures of cognitive function seemed to reverse after one year (Mulnard et al., 2000).

Of note, however, the results were not very different for the studies in our meta-analysis that had used an E_2. In women without dementia, the only positive results that remained significant were from two studies from one group, which administered a monthly bolus injection of E_2 for two to three months (Phillips and Sherwin, 1992; Sherwin, 1988). We could not replicate the positive effect of oral E_2 treatment (Linzmayer et al., 2001). It should be noted that the meta-analyses could not include some of the studies referred to earlier that had also used oral E_2 (Fedor-Freyberg, 1977; Hogervorst et al., 1999), either because data were not available or because criteria for inclusion were not met.

The mode of treatment could also be important. Our meta-analyses indicated that in women without dementia, transdermal treatment with E_2 (Duka et al., 2000; Dunkin et al., 2005; Polo-Kantola et al., 1998; Wolf et al., 1999) did not affect cognitive function. Although one study (Duka et al., 2000) reported positive effects of transdermal E_2 on visual memory and mental rotation tasks, these effects were not replicated in our meta-analyses and may be explained by baseline differences. In women with AD, transdermal E_2 improved cognition, but the effects were measured only up to eight weeks in one group (Asthana et al., 1999, 2001). The positive effects of transdermal E_2 in women with AD could be replicated in the meta-analyses. To our knowledge, bolus injections or oral E_2 administration have not been used in treatment studies of women with AD.

Bolus injections can increase E_2 levels 10-fold compared with transdermal treatment (Phillips and Sherwin, 1992; Sherwin, 1988). Transdermal E_2 also does not show the same increase in E_2 levels as most oral treatments. Oral E_2 was used in the studies that reported positive effects (Fedor-Freyberg, 1977; Hogervorst et al., 1999; Linzmayer et al., 2001).

As already mentioned, however, high E_2 levels are not necessarily related to better cognitive function. Although several treatment studies (e.g., Phillips and Sherwin, 1992; Wolf et al., 1999) reported a significant positive association between E_2 levels and verbal memory in women without AD, this association may not hold in women who are already afflicted with dementia. A post hoc analysis reported that in women with AD who had been treated with Premarin, high E_2 levels were not associated with better verbal recall (Thal et al., 2003). In another study, high E_2 levels were associated with worse delayed verbal recall and with a smaller hippocampus (Den Heijer et al., 2003). The association with hippocampal size is important, because a faster rate of hippocampal atrophy has been associated with AD (Jobst et al., 1992). Slightly but significantly higher levels of E_2 and/or estrone (E_1) have been found in women with AD (Cunningham et al., 2001; Geerlings et al., 2003; Hogervorst et al., 2003; Paoletti et al., 2004), and it is also possible that studies reporting lower levels in patients with AD may have included control subjects who were using HT (Manly et al., 2000), or the results may have been confounded by the use of estradiol assays with inadequate sensitivity (Hogervorst et al., 2003).

In addition, some treatment studies that could not be included in the meta-analyses suggested that after long-term treatment with E_2, the initial short-term positive effects may reverse. An early RCT in 1954 of institutionalized women with probable dementia reported that some cognitive functions declined after 18 months of treatment with an E_2 bolus injection and other hormones (Caldwell, 1954). We found similar effects in an unblinded study using oral E_2 and a progestagen in women without dementia who had severe menopausal complaints (Hogervorst et al., 1999). Hence, qualitative analyses suggest that the effects of E_2, similar to the effects of Premarin, may reverse after one year.

These findings, taken together, may indicate that the effects of both Premarin and E_2 are short-lived and do not exceed two to three months, after which some effects may even reverse. There are several theories of why this may be the case. Dominique Toran-Allerand has argued that receptor downregulation could be an important factor in explaining why continuous estrogen treatment used in most studies did not have a sustained positive effect on cognition (Toran-Allerand, 2004). This mechanism, although disputed (Gibbs, 2004), could occur when levels of estrogens are continuously elevated above endogenous levels. Different treatment regimens (e.g., low-dose estrogens given intermittently) could possibly prevent this outcome. In the animal studies reviewed in chapter 1, the use of low-dose or cyclical intermittent weekly treatment was more effective in sustaining cognitive function in ovariectomized rats than was continuous combination treatment. Although low-dose transdermal E_2 was not effective in improving cognition in humans without dementia, cyclical *weekly* combination treatment has not, to our knowledge, been tested in recently postmenopausal women.

With respect to the other types of estrogen, E_2 is the most potent of naturally occurring estrogens. Estrone (E_1) has less receptor affinity than E_2. An early RCT using E_1 for six months that was included in the meta-analyses (Hackman and Galbraith, 1977) showed only a trend on the Guild Memory Test in favor of treatment. In light of the E_2 results described earlier, it is likely that this effect would also reverse after a longer period of treatment. A longitudinal observational study found that high endogenous E_1 levels were associated with worse performance on some cognitive measures over time (Yaffe, Grady, et al., 1998). Estriol (E_3) has an even lower receptor affinity than E_1 and was reported to have only very small effects on vigilance and concentration in a three-month RCT (Vanhulle and Demol, 1976).

In sum, our meta-analyses showed that Premarin did not have any effects in women without dementia and had positive effects for only two to three months in women with dementia, after which the effects seemed to decrease or reverse. There was a similar short-term improvement after a bolus injection of E_2 in women without dementia and after transdermal E_2 application in women with AD.

Characteristics of Women Treated with HT
The Age of Women Treated: The Window-of-Opportunity Theory

Several of the RCTs that did not find positive effects of Premarin had enrolled women who were more than 65 years old (Binder et al., 2001; Goebel et al., 1995; Grady et al., 2002; Rapp et al., 2003) and for whom HT would normally not have been indicated. The reason for enrolling older women in the WHIMS study was pragmatic: below the age of 65, the risk for AD is very low. However, there may be a critical period for treatment to exert its positive effects. Animal studies suggest that HT may be effective in younger but not older females, and that a longer delay before initiating treatment (e.g., 10 instead of 3 months) after ovariectomy does not result in the favorable effects on brain function that are seen with early treatment (Gibbs in Henderson, 2004).

Although this is an attractive theory, and one that has received much attention, an RCT of asymptomatic, recently postmenopausal women less than 60 years old (average age, 53 years) also showed no improvement after treatment with CEE (Ditkoff et al., 1991). Although the tests used in this study may not have been sensitive to estrogenic effects, another study in women less than 62 years old (average age, 51 years) also found that CEE had no effect on performance on a verbal memory test (Shaywitz et al., 1999), the function believed to be most sensitive to estrogens (Sherwin, 1994).

On the other hand, qualitative analyses suggest that the studies showing positive results all included relatively young, postmenopausal women. The exception is the study by Polo-Kantola et al. (1998), which did not find any effects of transdermal E_2 and which included relatively young, naturally menopausal women (56 years old, on average) without a uterus (some of the older women had undergone ovariectomy, but only after their natural menopause). Conforming to the results of animal studies, this evidence thus suggests that an oral or bolus injection E_2 treatment is most effective in relatively young, recently postmenopausal women, but only for a two- to three-month period.

The strongest argument against the window-of-opportunity theory is that our meta-analyses showed that in women with AD (who were at least 10 years older than the women in the studies discussed in this section), both Premarin and transdermal E_2 had similarly positive but similarly short-lived (two to three months) effects. Hence, it seems more likely that positive effects, if they are found, are fleeting.

Surgical Menopause as a Risk Factor for Cognitive Decline

Our meta-analyses of women without dementia indicated that the significant effects of HT seemed to be limited to women who had undergone surgical menopause. A number of studies have shown a substantial drop in cognitive function after ovariectomy (Farrag et al., 2002; Nappi et al., 1999; Sherwin, 1988). This finding is in contrast to an observational study that could not find a drop in cognitive function with natural menopause (Henderson et al., 2003). Thus, it could be possible that surgical menopause is a risk factor for accelerated cognitive impairment, and ET would therefore be indicated for this group. One observational study (Verghese et al., 2000) reported better verbal memory and constructional abilities in surgically menopausal women using HT compared to age- and education-matched surgically menopausal women who had not used HT. Another observational study (File et al., 2002), however, found that surgically menopausal women who had an E_2 implant for about 10 years had worse long-term episodic memory and mental flexibility and more psychological and somatic menopausal symptoms than untreated surgically menopausal women. Menopausal symptoms did not explain the memory performance. These negative results could be in line with the findings of another group, which found an association between better fluency and HT use in younger (<58 years) surgically menopausal women but not older surgically or younger and older naturally menopausal women (Szklo et al., 1996). These findings also tie in with an observational study that indicated that former but not current users of HT were protected against AD (Zandi et al., 2002). Possibly treatment should be short (<1 year), but a short treatment period may have longer-lasting effects in protecting the brain against accelerated cognitive decline in surgically menopausal women. Alternatively, as suggested earlier, intermittent weekly treatment regimens may have longer-lasting positive effects.

The Treatment of Women Who Are Highly Symptomatic

It has been suggested that cognitive function appeared to improve in the earlier HT studies only because severe menopausal symptoms were alleviated (LeBlanc et al., 2001; Yaffe, Sawaya, et al.,1998). Our meta-analyses showed effects only in surgically menopausal women, and these women usually have perimenopausal symptoms of great severity. A more qualitative and detailed look at all studies that reported positive effects of E_2, with or without a pro-gestagen (Duka et al., 2000; Fedor-Freyberg, 1977; Hogervorst et al., 1999; Linz-mayer et al., 2001; Phillips and Sherwin, 1992; Sherwin, 1988), showed that most of these studies had included relatively young women, 48 to 58 years old, who were highly symptomatic and who usually went to a clinic for treat-ment of their symptoms. The only exception is the study by Duka et al. (2000), who measured elderly (65 years old), asymptomatic women, but the reported significant effects in this study could not be replicated in meta-analyses.

A few studies that statistically tested the hypothesis (e.g., Phillips and Sherwin, 1992; Wolf et al., 1999) reported that cognitive improvement was not mediated through an alleviation of depression or through improved sleep. Studies with phytoestrogens (Duffy et al., 2003; Kritz-Silverstein et al., 2003), which may act as estrogen agonists or antagonists, also reported improve-ments in cognitive function independent of menopausal symptoms.

HT lowers climacteric symptoms dramatically more than any other current treatment does. Some antidepressants (selective serotonin reuptake inhibitors, e.g., sertraline) have been used to lower flush frequency, but their efficacy is about half that of HT. Mood, sleep quality, and memory have also been re-ported to improve with this type of treatment (Goodnick et al., 2000), sug-gesting an association between symptoms and cognition independent of hor-monal mechanisms. To date, the question of whether cognition improves because of symptom alleviation has not been answered satisfactorily. More studies, using nonhormonal strategies to decrease menopausal symptoms, should also measure cognitive function to test this theory.

The Treatment of Women Who Are
Genetically at Risk for AD

There may be an interaction of HT with genetic factors, and HT could be more or less effective in women with particular polymorphisms. The presence of at least one APOE ε4 allele is approximately three times more common in individuals with AD (Hogervorst et al., 2002a). Although some observational studies noted that having an APOE ε4 allele seemed to be necessary for HT to protect against AD (Slooter et al., 1999; Tang et al., 1996), others found that cognitive decline was prevented only in women who were negative for the ε4 allele (Burkhardt et al., 2004; Yaffe, Haan, et al., 2000), and several reported that having the ε4 allele made no difference in risk reduction (Steffens et al.,

1999; Zandi et al., 2002). It is unclear whether discrepancies between these study results could potentially be explained by complex interactions with the APOE genotype and the age differences of the participants combined with the time of initiation of treatment or the duration of HT use (i.e., the effects of HT being protective in relatively recently menopausal women carrying the APOE ε4 allele).

We and others found that E_2 levels were slightly elevated in women with AD. Another possibility might be that women with AD have certain genotypes that predispose them to higher E_2 levels. Several genes are involved in E_2 metabolism and synthesis. The gene *CYP17* codes for an enzyme (cytochrome P450c17a) that helps regulate estrogen synthesis. The gene is located on chromosome 10 and has two alleles. A variation of this gene (polymorphism) can have a so-called A2 allele, which increases the amount of enzyme produced, which results in higher estrogen levels. The allele versions of this gene without this variation are called A1. Several studies have reported that homozygotes (persons who have both A2 allele versions: A2/A2) or heterozygotes (those with just one A2 allele: A2/A1) have increased E_2 levels compared with persons with both A1 alleles (A1/A1) (Sharp et al., 2004). It may be that increasing estrogen levels for women with the *CYP17* 5'-UTR gene polymorphism (the A2/A2 genotype), who may already have higher estrogen levels, could have negative effects. There may be an optimal dosage of estrogens for optimal effects on the brain, after which effects reverse and become negative.

P450(CYP)1B1 is also a key enzyme in the metabolism of E_2. The expression of cytochrome P450(CYP)1B1 leads to 4-hydroxylation of E_2, which results in a decrease in estrogenic activity (via the estrogen receptor). This produces a toxic metabolite that has been associated with DNA damage (Cecchin et al., 2004). DNA damage has been associated with pathology in AD (Smith, 2002). The Val432/Val allele variant is associated with higher 4-hydroxy E_2 levels than the Leu432 variant.

Last, the inactivation of reactive metabolites, such as catechol estrogens, is regulated by catechol-O-methyltransferase (COMT), which is regulated by the expression of COMT (Val108/158) Met. The COMT Met/Met polymorphism may be a risk factor when compared with the COMT Val/Val genotype in that reactive metabolites are not inactivated (Hamajima et al., 2001). If women have genotypes CYP17 A2, P450CYP1B1 Val432/Val, and COMT Met/Met and are then given HT, they might produce very high levels of toxic metabolites, which might put them at risk for dementia. To our knowledge, these risk polymorphisms have not been investigated in women with AD.

Socioeconomic Status, Lifelong Exposure to Estrogens, and Lifestyle Variables

Our review (Hogervorst et al., 2000) suggested that particularly vulnerable women with low levels of educational achievement and low SES (who are at additional risk for AD) may profit most from HT. These factors may be associated with lifelong exposure to health-related factors that affect estrogens indirectly. They may also contribute to lifelong exposure to estrogen levels directly, by affecting age at menarche and age at menopause. For instance, women of higher SES have been found to have an earlier age at menarche (Ayatollahi et al., 2002), which would give them a longer period of exposure to estrogens.

It is unclear, however, whether lifelong exposure, determined by a younger age at menarche and a later age at menopause, affects the risk for AD. One study reported a decreased risk for AD with a younger age at menarche (Paganini-Hill and Henderson, 1994), but several others did not (Balderischi et al., 1998; Kawas et al., 1996; Waring et al., 1999). Some studies found that a later age at menopause (Balderischi et al., 1998; McLay et al., 2003) protected against AD, but others could not repeat this finding (Kawas et al., 1996; Paganini-Hill and Henderson, 1994; Waring et al., 1999), and one study found the opposite (Geerlings et al., 2001). In that study, a longer reproductive period increased the risk for AD, but only in APOE ε4 carriers.

Lifestyle factors such as smoking may also interact with lifelong exposure and HT use. Smokers have an earlier menopause than nonsmokers (Kato et al., 1998) and are more likely to develop AD (Merchant et al., 1999). Smoking induces hepatic enzymes that metabolize estrogen (Meek and Finch, 1999), which would lower estrogen levels and also render HT less effective. One study (Brenner et al., 1994) that controlled for smoking found no protective effect of HT against AD. In contrast, another study (Lerner et al., 1997) reported a possible synergistic effect of smoking and HT in risk reduction.

Smokers also have lower levels of serum folate (Kim et al., 2004). We found that women with high levels of E_2 but who also had high levels of serum folate did not have Mini-Mental State Examination (MMSE) scores below the cutoff score for dementia when compared with women with low levels of serum folate (Hogervorst and Smith, 2002). Serum folate is inversely related to homocysteine, which in many studies was shown to be associated with vascular disease, cognitive decline, and AD, and with markers of dementia such as white matter disease, hippocampal atrophy, and cognitive dysfunction (Hogervorst et al., 2002). It is possible that giving women folic acid while they are using HT could protect against cognitive decline.

In sum, several lifestyle factors may modify the effect of HT, but the interactions may occur on different levels (including genetic subtypes) and may thus be very complicated. Artificial neural network techniques using higher-order interactions may prove helpful in assessing risks and benefits for the individual.

Women with AD Who Are Treated with Cholinesterase Inhibitors

Post hoc analyses of a tacrine treatment study (Schneider et al., 1996) suggested that women who were treated with a combination of HT and tacrine improved more in cognitive function than women not receiving ET, who had been randomly assigned to tacrine or to placebo. Although the number of women taking HT and tacrine was relatively small in this study, the results sparked new interest in the possible synergistic actions of HT and cholinesterase inhibitors such as tacrine, donepezil, and rivastigmine.

An RCT (Relkin et al., 2002) investigated 146 women with mild to moderate AD (mean age, 78; SD = 7 years) who had been using donepezil for an average of 51 weeks. A baseline was measured, and after six weeks women were randomly assigned to CEE or placebo. After 18 weeks no differences were seen between groups in cognitive performance (using the Alzheimer's Disease Assessment Scale–Cognitive subscale, or ADAS-Cog). A French group (Rigaud et al., 2003) investigated 117 women with mild to moderate AD (mean age, 76; SD = 7 years) who were all allocated to rivastigmine. In addition, women were randomly assigned to transdermal E_2 and an oral progesterone (Utrogestan) or placebo. No differences were seen after 12 or 28 weeks on several cognitive outcome measures (e.g., ADAS-Cog and MMSE) and the Instrumental Activities of Daily Life (IADL) score. Yoon et al. (2003) compared 55 women with AD (average age, 69 years) who had been given tacrine (n = 26) or CEE (26 were given CEE with MPA and 3 were given CEE by itself) in an RCT. There was a trend for the MMSE to improve after one month of both treatments; this trend stabilized at three months and seemed to reverse after six months. More detailed neuropsychological testing did not show any effects. Only the IADL score was better after HT when compared with tacrine after six months.

In sum, none of these studies showed that HT had beneficial effects on cognitive function over those of cholinesterase inhibitors when tested in comparison or in combination treatment. After the negative results of traditional estrogen-based treatment, more research is now directed toward finding potential alternatives for treating menopausal complaints and preventing dementia.

Alternatives to Treat Menopausal Complaints and Cognitive Dysfunction
Selective Estrogen Receptor Modulators

Selective estrogen receptor modulators (SERMs) were thought to be a good alternative to traditional HT, and several large trials of SERMs are still ongoing. SERMs can act as antagonists but also as estrogen agonists, and were thought to prevent or treat breast and endometrial cancer by acting as estrogen antagonists and to prevent osteoporosis and CHD by acting as estrogen agonists.

Large randomized trials found that women who took raloxifene or tamoxifen for four years reduced their risk of breast cancer by 65 percent or 50 percent, respectively. However, guidelines from the U.S. Preventive Services Task Force (Kinsinger et al., 2002) reported that the risks of tamoxifen and raloxifene could outweigh the benefits. Studies indicated that both SERMs increased the risk for thromboembolic disease, as well as having undesirable side effects such as hot flushes. In addition, although women with breast cancer who took tamoxifen for five years were less likely to have a recurrence, those who continued to take the drug for another five years had a greater risk of recurrent cancer than those who stopped. Last, tamoxifen, but not raloxifene, was reported to substantially increase the risk of endometrial cancer.

To date, the effects of SERMs on cognitive function do not seem overwhelming. Similar to CEE with MPA, their association with thromboembolic disease and stroke could indicate that longer treatment produces a risk for cognitive decline and dementia. In this line, in an observational study of 1,163 women, tamoxifen use (for an average of five years) was associated with small negative effects on cognitive function (narrative writing), with users also having more memory complaints than never users (Paganini-Hill and Clark, 2000).

Raloxifene also did not prevent cognitive decline in an RCT after one year in 143 postmenopausal women (Nickelsen et al., 1999). The Memory Assessment Clinics (MAC) battery and the Walter Reed Performance Assessment Battery showed no difference after 12 months of treatment. The only significant

difference observed was a slight increase in performance favoring the raloxifene, 120 mg/day group, in an assessment of verbal memory on the MAC battery after one month of treatment. In the Multiple Outcomes of Raloxifene
Evaluation (MORE) trial (Yaffe et al., 2001), 7,478 postmenopausal women
with osteoporosis (mean age, 66 years) were randomly assigned to receive
raloxifene (60 mg or 120 mg) or placebo daily for three years. There were no
differences in cognitive function between groups overall. There were trends
for subgroups that showed greater cognitive decline to do less so in the combined raloxifene group than placebo users on the two tests of verbal memory
and attention. Newly reported or worsening hot flushes did not negatively
influence test scores or the effect of treatment on test performance.

Tibolone

Tibolone has estrogenic, progestagenic, or androgenic metabolites and exhibits tissue-specific hormonal effects. Tibolone also lowers sex hormone–
binding globulin, which increases bioavailable E_2 and testosterone levels.
Women treated with tibolone reported significant reductions in vaginal dryness and flushes (for a review, see Davis, 2002).

An observational study included 25 postmenopausal women, 54 to 66 years
old, who had been taking tibolone (Livial, 2.5 mg/day) for approximately
10 years and matched them with 25 non-HT-using women for age, years since
menopause, IQ, years of secondary education, occupation, and anxiety and
depression scores. Women taking Livial reported to be less clumsy and to feel
less stressful after a stressful test. They also had better semantic memory (category generation task), but not episodic memory. On the other hand, women
in the tibolone group also performed significantly worse on a sustained attention task and a planning task, which are associated with frontal lobe function (Fluck et al., 2002).

The effects of tibolone on cognitive function were also not found to be
greater than those of CEE combined with a progestagen or of E_2 combined with
norethisterone acetate. These studies did not include a placebo group or a control group, which makes it difficult to assess whether improvements could be
attributed to therapy.

A single-blind study comparing CEE and MPA with tibolone in post-
menopausal women showed a small improvement in cognitive function with
CEE after three months, but no additional improvement at six months.
Tibolone showed no effects and did not increase estradiol levels (Pan et al.,

2003). In another study, 38 perimenopausal symptomatic women were given either CEE and a progestagen (norgestrel) for the last 12 days of each 28-day cycle or tibolone for 28 days. There were no significant differences in changes from baseline between the two treatments. For both groups combined there were significant improvements compared with baseline in vasomotor symptoms in the first month, and improvements in anxiety, sleep, memory, and somatic dysfunction by the second and third months, but no improvement in depression scores. In this study, alleviation of memory problems was related to an improvement in vasomotor symptoms but was independent of depression (Ross et al., 1999). Another six-month, single-blind study of 22 postmenopausal women 51 to 57 years old investigated the difference between continuous combined estradiol plus norethisterone acetate (Kliogest) and tibolone (Livial). Fourteen patients completed the study. Libido (but not mood) was improved after both treatments equally. Recognition memory improved after treatment with Kliogest, but not after treatment with Livial. Both drugs resulted in equal improvements on reaction time and accuracy of performance of categorical semantic memory (Albertazzi et al., 2000). The latter effects could be attributed to learning effects and hence should be regarded with caution.

In sum, these preliminary results of studies do not suggest that tibolone would be an alternative to traditional HT regimens.

Phytoestrogens

Phytoestrogens are naturally occurring plant estrogens. They are abundant in soy products such as tofu but also occur in grains, fruits, and other vegetables. They have estrogenic and antiestrogenic properties and act through a weak binding to the estrogen receptor. Phytoestrogens may reduce the risk for cancer and also cardiovascular disease (for a review, see Kris-Etherton et al., 2002). The cardioprotective effect could indicate that they have a better long-term profile in protecting against age-related cognitive decline. In addition, phytoestrogens were found to exert antioxidant-like effects on hippocampal neurons that had been exposed to glutamate and β-amyloid. However, they did not show the same neurotrophic effects that estradiol did (Zhao et al., 2002). One uncontrolled study of 127 women with an average age of 57 years (without a placebo arm, but controls received no treatment) reported that CEE plus MPA and the equivalent of 100 mg of isoflavones improved performance on the MMSE and a speed-of-information-processing task after three months. CEE had superior effects over isoflavones on a delayed re-call task. There was no change in menopausal symptoms or well-being (Woo et al., 2003). A three-month RCT of 33 postmenopausal women 50 to 65 years old indicated that those receiving a soya supplement (60 mg/day of total isoflavone equivalents) had significantly greater improvement in recall of pic-tures, on a sustained attention task, in learning rule reversals, and on a plan-ning task than those given a placebo. Improvements were independent of any changes in menopausal symptoms, mood, or sleepiness (Duffy et al., 2003). In a six-month RCT involving 53 postmenopausal women 55 to 74 years old, however, only one out of five cognitive functions showed a small improve-ment (Kritz-Silverstein et al., 2003). Women who had been given 110 mg/day of total isoflavones showed greater improvement only on category fluency and nonsignificant improvements on two other tests of verbal memory and Trails B. In an RCT of 12 months, the equivalent of 99 mg/day of isoflavones had no effect on a wide range of cognitive function, including tests of verbal mem-ory (Kreijkamp-Kaspers et al., 2005). Tentatively, these findings seem to be in line with E_2 treatment findings that suggest that hormones may have posi-tive effects for up to two to three months, after which their effects plateau, and may reverse after 12 months.

Long-term high phytoestrogen intake is not necessarily without risk. The Honolulu Heart Study, an observational study, found that men (and their wives) who reported consuming tofu more than twice a week had a higher risk of dementia and lower cognitive function at an older age than those who con-sumed less (White et al., 2000). However, different foods may have different effects, and self-reported dietary assessment can be unreliable. Future obser-vational studies should include serum or saliva phytoestrogen levels.

Androgens: Testosterone, DHEA, DHEAS

One (Sherwin, 1988) of the two RCTs that showed significant effects in our meta-analyses had also employed intramuscular testosterone treatment using a crossover design for three months. The effects of testosterone plus E_2 on two tests of short-term memory, a test of long-term memory, and a test of log-ical reasoning were not larger than the effects of E_2 (or testosterone) alone. In a study of 35 healthy postmenopausal women who were already using CEE, CEE was replaced by 0.625 mg of oral esterified estrogen (EE), which was given either alone or in combination with 1.25 mg of oral methyltestosterone (meT) according to a two eight-week crossover design. Adding meT significantly improved scores on a test of complex information processing but not on other tests (Regestein et al., 2001). In another four-month study (Wisniewski et al., 2002), estrogen alone or in combination with oral meT was investigated in postmenopausal women for four months. Women receiving estrogen and meT maintained a steady level of performance on only one out of four tests (the Building Memory task), whereas those who received estrogen alone showed a decrease in performance on this test. A crossover study of only three days compared transdermal testosterone with placebo (n = 12) and transdermal E_2 with placebo (n = 12) in relatively young, postmenopausal women (average age, 58 years). The authors reported that E_2 impaired divergent thinking and improved convergent thinking, motor perseveration, and verbal memory. Testosterone's effects were opposite those of E_2 in that it improved performance on some divergent thinking tasks (Krug et al., 2003).

These studies were all relatively small and of relatively short duration. Of note, testosterone, similar to estrogens, can increase the risk for breast cancer, and high levels of testosterone have been associated with cardiovascular disease in women (Wu and von Eckardstein, 2003). Thus, it does not seem likely that long-term treatment with testosterone will have additional benefits and fewer risks than treatment with E_2. There is also little evidence to suggest that DHEAS or DHEA has positive effects on cognitive function in postmenopausal women (Huppert and Van Niekerk, 2001; Wolf, 2003).

Conclusions
Treatment Regimens

We have reviewed studies to investigate whether there is a case for HT to maintain cognitive function in postmenopausal women. The largest study to date, the WHIMS study, which showed negative effects, had added MPA to the estrogen treatment. This regimen may have more negative effects on cardiovascular and cholinergic functions, which may negatively affect cognitive decline, particularly after a longer period of treatment. The WHIMS estrogen-only arm, however, still showed a trend toward an increased risk for dementia. Our meta-analyses showed that the synthetic estrogens used in the WHI study (Premarin) never had positive effects on cognitive function in comparison with a placebo in women without dementia.

Qualitative analyses showed that a bolus injection or oral administration of estradiol (E_2), with or without different progestagens, produced a positive effect. Transdermal E_2 treatment did not seem to be effective in women without dementia. Treatment success seemed to be short-lived (two to three months), however, and some positive effects reversed after one year, similar to the effects of Premarin.

The Characteristics of Women Treated

The studies that reported positive effects of HT all included relatively young, recently postmenopausal women, generally less than 60 years old. Animal studies suggest that age may be an important factor in treatment. However, Premarin also never showed a positive effect in studies that included younger postmenopausal women. The other fact is that both Premarin and transdermal E_2 did have some positive effects in women with dementia for a short period (two to three months). These women were, on average, 15 years past menopause, which indicates that age at treatment may not be the most important factor.

To further investigate this, we did statistical analyses on the RCT studies of women without dementia using logistic regression techniques and found that the duration of the study was the main determinant of outcome. Studies with positive effects had a mean duration of three months, whereas studies with no effects had an average duration of 7.6 months ($P < 0.05$). Negative studies had an average duration of 76 months. Participant age contributed non-significantly to study outcome ($P = 0.88$); the average age in the studies reporting positive effects was 64 years and in the negative studies it was 65 years.

The evidence thus suggests that the initial short-term positive effects on cognitive function reverse after a year of treatment with Premarin in women with (Mulnard et al., 2000) and without dementia (Rapp et al., 2003), but also after a bolus injection of E_2 in women with probable dementia (Caldwell, 1954), after a bolus injection in surgically menopausal women (File et al., 2002), and after oral E_2 in women without dementia (Hogervorst et al., 1999). These results, taken together with the findings discussed earlier, seem to indicate that the effects of both Premarin and E_2 are relatively small (they are not always measured, depending on the cognitive test used), probably short-lived, and tend to reverse after one year.

It is unclear whether surgically menopausal women are at additional risk for cognitive decline, but in light of the information presented in this chapter, perhaps treatment should be limited to one year, or, alternatively, cyclical intermittent weekly combination treatment should be considered. In addition, qualitative analyses showed that all studies with positive effects included women with severe menopausal symptoms. The extent to which symptom alleviation improves cognitive function is unclear, but comparative studies using selective serotonin reuptake inhibitors could shed more light on this question.

Possibly other characteristics of women, such as genetic differences or lifestyle variables, could determine a different outcome. It is unclear whether lifelong exposure to estrogen levels makes a difference to the risk of dementia. The use of artificial neural network strategies, which can handle complex interactions on different levels, could aid in assessing the probable risks and benefits of treatment for the individual.

Alternative Treatments

We reviewed the evidence for possible effects of alternative treatments on cognitive function. Contrary to expectations, SERMs were found to induce an increased risk for cancers and cerebrovascular disease, which, similar to treatment with Premarin and MPA, could indicate that longer treatment produces a risk for cognitive decline and dementia. The effects of SERMs on cognitive function were either negative or very small. The small studies of tibolone and testosterone that we reviewed had methodological problems (no inclusion of a placebo group, but instead a comparison with Premarin or E_2). The effects on cognitive function of these treatments appear not to be greater than those of traditional estrogen treatment. The results of phytoestrogen trials may suggest that this group's effects, like those of traditional estrogen treatment, are positive for up to three months, and then may reverse after one year.

In sum, currently there is no evidence to indicate that long-term (longer than one year) treatment with HT (Premarin or other types of HT, such as estradiol or phytoestrogens) would prevent cognitive decline in women with or without dementia. In general, the effects of HT on cognition are short-lived (two to three months) and seem to reverse after one year. There is little evidence that effects will be positive with a longer period of treatment in younger, recently postmenopausal women. Progestagens other than MPA have not shown additional negative effects on cognitive function, but these short-term studies were all done in relatively young, symptomatic women, and it is unclear what the effects of a longer duration of treatment would be. It is also unclear whether women who have undergone surgical menopause or who have excessive symptoms can profit from short-term treatment for a longer period. Whether symptoms mediate cognition improvement deserves further investigation, possibly by using new-generation antidepressants. Observational studies may have been confounded by a biased recall and by healthy lifestyle patterns, incorporating exercise and a healthy diet, in HT users. These factors affect both the risk for cardiovascular or cerebrovascular disease and the risk for dementia. Currently, no alternative HT therapies are available that will reverse cognitive decline in elderly women. However, we recommend large RCTs to investigate the effect of cyclical intermittent weekly combination treatment of E_2 with a progestagen other than MPA in women who have recently become menopausal.

REFERENCES

Albertazzi P, Natale V, Barbolini C, et al. 2000. The effect of tibolone versus continuous combined norethisterone acetate and oestradiol on memory, libido and mood of postmenopausal women: a pilot study. Maturitas 36:223–29.

Amaducci LA, Fratiglioni L, Rocca WA, et al. 1986. Risk factors for clinically diagnosed Alzheimer's disease: a case-control study of an Italian population. Neurology 36:922–31.

Anderson GL, Limacher M, Assaf AR, et al. 2004. Effects of conjugated equine estrogen in postmenopausal women with hysterectomy: the Women's Health Initiative randomized controlled trial. JAMA 291:1769–71.

Asthana S, Baker LD, Craft S, et al. 2001. High-dose estradiol improves cognition for women with AD: results of a randomized study. Neurology 57:605–12.

Asthana S, Craft S, Baker LD, et al. 1999. Cognitive and neuroendocrine response to transdermal estrogen in postmenopausal women with AD: results of a placebo-controlled, double-blind pilot study. Psychoneuroendocrinology 24:657–77.

Ayatollahi SM, Dowlatabadi E, Ayatollahi SA. 2002. Age at menarche in Iran. Ann Hum Biol 29:355-62.

Balderischi M, DiCarlo A, Lepore V, et al. 1998. Estrogen-replacement therapy and Alzheimer's disease in the Italian Longitudinal Study on Aging. Neurology 50:996–1002.

Barrett-Connor E. 1998. Rethinking estrogen and the brain. J Am Geriatr Soc 46:918–20.

Barrett-Connor E, Goodman-Gruen D. 1999. Cognitive function and endogenous sex hormones in older women. J Am Geriatr Soc 47:1289–93.

Barrett-Connor E, Kritz-Silverstein D. 1999. Gender differences in cognitive function with age: the Rancho Bernardo Study. J Am Geriatr Soc 47:159–64.

Binder EF, Schechtman KB, Birge SJ, et al. 2001. Effects of hormone replacement therapy on cognitive performance in elderly women. Maturitas 38:137–46.

Borenstein-Graves A, White E, Koepsell TD, et al. 1990. A case-control study of Alzheimer's disease. Ann Neurol 28:766–74.

Brenner DE, Kukull WA, Stergachis A, et al. 1994. Postmenopausal estrogen replacement therapy and the risk of Alzheimer's disease: a population-based case-control study. Am J Epidemiol 140:262–67.

Broe GA, Henderson AS, Creasey H, et al. 1990. A case-control study of Alzheimer's disease in Australia. Neurology 40:1698–1707.

Burkhardt MS, Foster JK, Laws SM, et al. 2004. Oestrogen replacement therapy may improve memory functioning in the absence of APOE epsilon4. J Alzheimers Dis 6:221–28.

Caldwell BM. 1954. An evaluation of psychological effects of sex hormone administration in aged women. II. Results of therapy after 18 months. J Gerontol 9:168–74.

Carlson LE, Sherwin BB. 1998. Steroid hormones, memory and mood in a healthy elderly population. Psychoneuroendocrinology 30:583–603.

Cecchin E, Russo A, Campagnutta E, et al. 2004. Lack of association of CYP1 B1*3 polymorphism and ovarian cancer in a Caucasian population. Int J Biol Markers 19:160–63.

Cerhan JR, Folsom AR, Mortimer JA, et al. 1998. Correlates of cognitive function in middle aged adults. Gerontology 44:95–105.

Cunningham CJ, Sinnott M, Denihan A, et al. 2001. Endogenous sex hormone levels in postmenopausal women with AD. J Clin Endocrinol Metab 86:1099–1103.

Davis SR. 2002. The effects of tibolone on mood and libido. Menopause 9:162–70.

Den Heijer T, Geerlings MI, Hofman A, et al. 2003. Higher estrogen levels are not associated with larger hippocampi and better memory performance. Arch Neurol 60:213–20.

Ditkoff EC, Crary WG, Cristo M, et al. 1991. Estrogen improves psychological function in asymptomatic postmenopausal women. Obstet Gynecol 78:991–95.

Drake EB, Henderson VW, Stanczyk FZ, et al. 2000. Associations between circulating sex steroid hormones and cognition in normal elderly women. Neurology 54:599–603.

Duffy R, Wiseman H, File SE. 2003. Improved cognitive function in postmenopausal women after 12 weeks of consumption of a soya extract containing isoflavones. Pharmacol Biochem Behav 75:721–29.

Duka T, Tasker R, McGowan JF. 2000. The effects of 3-week estrogen hormone replacement on cognition in elderly healthy females. Psychopharmacology 149:129–39.

Dunkin J, Rasgon N, Wagner-Steh K, et al. 2005. Reproductive events modify the effects of estrogen replacement therapy on cognition in healthy postmenopausal women. Psychoneuroendocrinology 30:284–96.

Farrag AK, Khedr EM, Abdel-Aleem H, et al. 2002. Effect of surgical menopause on cognitive functions. Dement Geriatr Cogn Disord 13:193–98.

Fedor-Freyberg P. 1977. The influence of estrogens on the well-being and mental performance in climacteric and postmenopausal women. Acta Obstet Gynecol Scand 64:12–20.

File SE, Heard JE, Rymer J. 2002. Trough oestradiol levels associated with cognitive impairment in post-menopausal women after 10 years of oestradiol implants. Psychopharmacology (Berl) 161:107–12.

Fillit HM, Ashby D, Weinreb H, et al. 1986. Estrogen levels in postmenopausal women with senile dementia–Alzheimer's type (SDAT) are significantly lower than matched controls. Soc Neurosci Abstr 12:A529.11.

Fluck E, File SE, Rymer J. 2002. Cognitive effects of 10 years of hormone-replacement therapy with tibolone. J Clin Psychopharmacol 22:62–67.

Geerlings MI, Launer LJ, de Jong FH, et al. 2003. Endogenous estradiol and risk of dementia in women and men: the Rotterdam Study. Ann Neurol 53:607–15.

Geerlings MI, Ruitenberg A, Witteman JC, et al. 2001. Reproductive period and risk of dementia in postmenopausal women. JAMA 285:1475–81.

Gibbs R. 2004. E-mail communication to E. Hogervorst, November 11.

Goebel JA, Birge SJ, Price SC, et al. 1995. Estrogen replacement therapy and postural stability in the elderly. Am J Otol 16:470–74.

Goodnick PJ, Chaudry T, Artadi J, et al. 2000. Women's issues in mood disorders. Expert Opin Pharmacother 1:903–16.

Grady D, Yaffe K, Kristof M, et al. 2002. Effect of postmenopausal hormone therapy on cognitive function: the Heart and Estrogen/Progestin Replacement Study. Am J Med 113:543–48.

Hackman BW, Galbraith D. 1977. Six month study of oestrogen therapy with piperazine oestrone sulphate and its effects on memory. Curr Med Res Opin 4:21–27.

Hamajima N, Matsuo K, Tajima K, et al. 2001. Limited association between a catechol-O-methyltransferase (COMT) polymorphism and breast cancer risk in Japan. Int J Clin Oncol 6:13–18.

Henderson VW. 2004. Hormone therapy and Alzheimer's disease: benefit or harm? Expert Opin Pharmacother 5:389–406.

Henderson VW, Guthrie JR, Dudley EC, et al. 2003. Estrogen exposures and memory at midlife: a population-based study of women. Neurology 60:1369–71.

Henderson VW, Paganini-Hill A, Emanuel CK, et al. 1994. Estrogen replacement therapy in older women: comparisons between Alzheimer's disease cases and nondemented control subjects. Arch Neurol 51:896–900.

Henderson VW, Paganini-Hill A, Miller BL, et al. 2000. Estrogen for Alzheimer's disease in women. Neurology 54:295–301.

Heyman A, Wilkinson WE, Stafford JA, et al. 1984. Alzheimer's disease: a study of epidemiological aspects. Ann Neurol 15:335–41.

Hogervorst E, Bandelow S, Hart J Jr, et al. 2004. Telephone word-list recall tested in the rural aging and memory study: two parallel versions for the TICS-M. Int J Geriatr Psychiatry 19:875–80.

Hogervorst E, Boshuisen M, Riedel WJ, et al. 1999. The effect of hormone replacement therapy on cognitive function in elderly women. Psychoneuroendocrinology 24: 43–68.

Hogervorst E, De Jager C, Budge MM, et al. 2004. Serum levels of estradiol and testosterone and performance in different cognitive domains in healthy elderly men and women. Psychoneuroendocrinology 29:405–21.

Hogervorst E, Mendes Ribeiro H, Molyneux A, et al. 2002. Serum homocysteine, cerebrovascular risk factors and white matter low attenuation on CT scans in patients with post-mortem confirmed AD. Arch Neurol 59:787–93.

Hogervorst E, Smith AD. 2002. The interaction of serum folate and estradiol levels in Alzheimer's disease. Neuroendocrinol Lett 23:155–60.

Hogervorst E, Williams J, Budge M, et al. 2000. The nature of the effect of female gonadal hormone replacement therapy on cognitive function in post-menopausal women: a meta-analysis. Neuroscience 101:485–512.

Hogervorst E, Williams J, Combrinck M, et al. 2003. Measuring serum oestradiol in women with Alzheimer's disease: the importance of the sensitivity of the assay method. Eur J Endocrinol 148:67–72.

Hogervorst E, Yaffe K, Richards M, et al. 2002a. Hormone replacement therapy for cognitive function in postmenopausal women. Cochrane Database Syst Rev 3:CD003122.

Hogervorst E, Yaffe K, Richards M, et al. 2002b. Hormone replacement therapy to maintain cognitive function in women with dementia. Cochrane Database Syst Rev 3: CD003799.

Huppert FA, Van Niekerk JK. 2001. Dehydroepiandrosterone (DHEA) supplementation for cognitive function. Cochrane Database Syst Rev 2:CD000304.

Jacobs DM, Tang M-X, Stern Y, et al. 1998. Cognitive function in non-demented older women who took estrogen after menopause. Neurology 30:368–73.

Jobst KA, Smith AD, Szatmari M, et al. 1992. Detection in life of confirmed Alzheimer's disease using a simple measurement of medial temporal lobe atrophy by computed tomography. Lancet 340:1179–83.

Kato I, Toniolo P, Akhmedkhanov A, et al. 1998. Prospective study of factors influencing the onset of natural menopause. J Clin Epidemiol 51:1271–76.

Kawas C, Resnick S, Morrison A, et al. 1996. A prospective study of estrogen replacement therapy and the risk of developing Alzheimer's disease. Neurology 48:1517–21.

Kim SH, Ensunsa JL, Zhu QY, et al. 2004. An 18-month follow-up study on the influence of smoking on blood antioxidant status of teenage girls in comparison with adult male smokers in Korea. Nutrition 20:437–44.

Kinsinger LS, Harris R, Woolf SH, et al. 2002. Chemoprevention of breast cancer: a summary of the evidence for the U.S. Preventive Services Task Force. Ann Intern Med 137: 59–69.

Kreijkamp-Kaspers S, Kok L, Grobbee DE, et al. 2005. Effect of soy protein containing isoflavones on cognitive function, bone mineral density, and plasma lipids in postmenopausal women: a randomized, controlled trial. Obstet Gynecol Surv 60:41–43.

Kris-Etherton PM, Hecker KD, Bonanome A, et al. 2002. Bioactive compounds in foods: their role in the prevention of cardiovascular disease and cancer. Am J Med 113: 71S–88S.

Kritz-Silverstein D, Von Muhlen D, Barrett-Connor E, et al. 2003. Isoflavones and cognitive function in older women: the Soy and Postmenopausal Health in Aging (SOPHIA) study. Menopause 10:196–202.

Krug R, Molle M, Dodt C, et al. 2003. Acute influences of estrogen and testosterone on divergent and convergent thinking in postmenopausal women. Neuropsychopharmacology 28:1538–45.

Launer LJ, Andersen K, Dewy ME, et al. 1999. Rates and risk factors for dementia and Alzheimer's disease. Neurology 1:78–84.

LeBlanc ES, Janowsky J, Chan BK, et al. 2001. Hormone replacement therapy and cognition: systematic review and meta-analysis. JAMA 285:1489–99.

Lerner A, Koss E, Debanne S, et al. 1997. Smoking and oestrogen replacement therapy as protective factors against AD. Lancet 349:403–4.

Linzmayer L, Semlitsch HV, Saletu B, et al. 2001. Double-blind, placebo-controlled psychometric studies on the effects of a combined estrogen-progestin regimen versus estrogen alone on performance, mood and personality of menopausal syndrome patients. Arzneimittelforschung 51:238–45.

Lokkegaard E, Pedersen AT, Laursen P, et al. 2002. The influence of hormone replacement therapy on the aging-related change in cognitive performance: analysis based on a Danish cohort study. Maturitas 42:209–18.

Manly JJ, Merchant CA, Jacobs DM, et al. 2000. Endogenous estrogen levels and Alzheimer's disease among postmenopausal women. Neurology 54:833–37.

Matthews K, Cauley J, Yaffe K, et al. 1999. Estrogen replacement therapy and cognitive decline in older community women. J Am Geriatr Soc 47:518–23.

Matthews KA, Kuller LH, Wing RR, et al. 1996. Prior to use of estrogen replacement therapy: are users healthier than nonusers? Am J Epidemiol 143:971–78.

McKhann G, Drachmann D, Folstein M, et al. 1984. Clinical diagnosis of Alzheimer's disease: report of the NINCDS-ADRDA work group under the auspices of Department of Health and Human Services Task Force on Alzheimer's Disease. Neurology 34:939–44.

McLay RN, Maki PM, Lyketsos CG. 2003. Nulliparity and late menopause are associated with decreased cognitive decline. J Neuropsychiatry Clin Neurosci 15:161–67.

Meek MD, Finch GL. 1999. Diluted mainstream cigarette smoke condensates activate estrogen receptor and aryl hydrocarbon receptor–mediated gene transcription. Environ Res 80:9–17.

Merchant C, Tang M-X, Albert S, et al. 1999. The influence of smoking on the risk of Alzheimer's disease. Neurology 52:1408–12.

Mortel KF, Meyer JS. 1995. Lack of postmenopausal estrogen replacement therapy and the risk of dementia. J Neuropsychiatry Clin Neurosci 7:334–37.

Mulnard RA, Cotman CW, Kawas C, et al. 2000. Estrogen replacement therapy for treatment of mild to moderate Alzheimer's disease. JAMA 283:1007–15.

Nappi RE, Sinforiani E, Mauri M, et al. 1999. Memory functioning at menopause: impact of age in ovariectomized women. Gynecol Obstet Invest 47:29–36.

Nickelsen T, Lufkin EG, Riggs BL, et al. 1999. Raloxifene hydrochloride, a selective estrogen receptor modulator: safety assessment of effects on cognitive function and mood in postmenopausal women. Psychoneuroendocrinology 24:115–28.

Paganini-Hill A, Clark LJ. 2000. Preliminary assessment of cognitive function in breast cancer patients treated with tamoxifen. Breast Cancer Res Treat 64:165–76.

Paganini-Hill A, Henderson VW. 1994. Estrogen deficiency and risk of Alzheimer's disease in women. Am J Epidemiol 140:256–61.

Paganini-Hill A, Henderson VW. 1996. The effect of hormone replacement therapy lipoprotein cholesterol levels and other factors on a clock drawing task in older women. J Am Geriatr Soc 44:818–22.

Pan H-A, Wang S-T, Pai M-C, et al. 2003. Cognitive function variations in postmenopausal women treated with continuous, combined HT or tibolone: a comparison. J Reprod Med 48:375–80.

Paoletti AM, Congia S, Lello S, et al. 2004. Low androgenization index in elderly women and elderly men with Alzheimer's disease. Neurology 62:301–3.

Petitti DB, Buckwalter JG, Crooks VC, et al. 2002. Prevalence of dementia in users of hormone replacement therapy as defined by prescription data. J Gerontol A Biol Sci Med Sci 57:M532–38.

Phillips SM, Sherwin BB. 1992. Effects of estrogen on memory function in surgically menopausal women. Psychoneuroendocrinology 17:485–95.

Polo-Kantola P, Portin R, Polo O, et al. 1998. The effect of short-term estrogen replacement therapy on cognition: a randomized double-blind, cross-over trial in postmenopausal women. Obstet Gynecol 91:459–66.

Rapp SR, Espeland MA, Shumaker SA, et al. 2003. Effect of estrogen plus progestin on global cognitive function in postmenopausal women: the Women's Health Initiative Memory Study: a randomized controlled trial. JAMA 289:2663–72.

Regestein QR, Friebely J, Shifren J, et al. 2001. Neuropsychological effects of methyltestosterone in women using menopausal hormone replacement. J Womens Health Gend Based Med 10:671–76.

Relkin N, McRae T, Reuss V, et al. 2002. Estrogen does not enhance the efficacy of donepezil in the treatment of women with Alzheimer's disease. Paper presented at the 8th International Conference on AD and Related Disorders (p. 53). Stockholm, Sweden.

Rigaud AS, Andre G, Vellas B, et al. 2003. No additional benefit of HT on response to rivastigmine in menopausal women with AD. Neurology 60:148–49.

Ross LA, Alder EM, Cawood EH, et al. 1999. Psychological effects of hormone replacement therapy: a comparison of tibolone and a sequential estrogen therapy. Psychosom Obstet Gynaecol 20:88–96.

Rymer J, Wilson R, Ballard K. 2003. Making decisions about hormone replacement therapy. BMJ 326:322–26.

Sarrel PM. 1989. Effects of ovarian steroids on the cardiovascular system. In *The Circulation of the Female from the Cradle to the Grave,* ed. J Ginsberg, 112–40. Carnford, U.K.: Parthenon Publishing.

Schneider LS, Farlow MR, Henderson VW, et al. 1996. Effects of estrogen replacement therapy in response to tacrine in patients with Alzheimer's disease. Neurology 46:1580–84.

Seshadri S, Zornberg G, Derby LE, et al. 2001. Postmenopausal estrogen replacement therapy and the risk of Alzheimer disease. Arch Neurol 58:435–40.

Sharp L, Cardy AH, Cotton SC, et al. 2004. *CYP17* gene polymorphisms: prevalence and associations with hormone levels and related factors. A HuGE review. Am J Epidemiol 160:729–40.

Shaywitz SE, Shaywitz BE, Pugh KR, et al. 1999. Effects of estrogen on brain activation patterns in postmenopausal women during working memory tasks. JAMA 281:1197–202.

Sherwin BB. 1988. Estrogen and/or androgen replacement therapy and cognitive functioning in surgically menopausal women. Psychoneuroendocrinology 13:345–57.

Sherwin BB. 1994. Estrogenic effects on memory in women. Ann N Y Acad Sci 743: 213–30.

Shumaker SA, Legault C, Rapp SR, et al. 2003. Estrogen plus progestin and the incidence of dementia and mild cognitive impairment in postmenopausal women. JAMA 289:2651–62.

Slooter AJC, Bronzova J, Witteman JCM, et al. 1999. Estrogen use and early onset Alzheimer's disease: a population based study. J Neurol Neurosurg Psychiatry 67: 779–81.

Smith AD. 2002. Homocysteine, B vitamins, and cognitive deficit in the elderly. Am J Clin Nutr 75:785–86.

Steffens DC, Noron MC, Plassman BL, et al. 1999. Enhanced cognitive performance with estrogen use in nondemented community dwelling older women. J Am Geriatr Soc 47:1171–75.

Szklo M, Cerhan J, Diez-Roux AV, et al. 1996. Estrogen replacement therapy and cognitive functioning in the Atherosclerotic Risk in Communities (ARIC) study. Am J Epidemiol 144:1048–57.

Tang M-X, Jacobs D, Stern Y, et al. 1996. Effect of estrogen during menopause on risk and age of onset of Alzheimer's disease. Lancet 348:429–32.

Thal LJ, Thomas RG, Mulnard R, et al. 2003. Estrogen levels do not correlate with improvement in cognition. Arch Neurol 60:209–12.

Toran-Allerand D. 2004. Oral remarks at a meeting, Neurobiology and Neuroendocrinology of Aging, Bregenz, Austria, July 18–23.

Vanhulle G, Demol R. 1976. A double-blind study into the influences of estriol on a number of psychological tests in postmenopausal women. In Consensus on Menopausal Research, ed. PA van Keep, RB Greenblatt, M Albeaux-Fernet, 94–99. London: MTP Press.

Verghese J, Kuslansky G, Katz M. 2000. Surgically menopausal women on estrogen have better cognitive performance. Neurology 54:A210–11.

Wang PN, Liao SQ, Liu RS, et al. 2000. Effects of estrogen on cognition, mood, and cerebral blood flow in AD. Neurology 54:2061–66.

Waring SC, Rocca WA, Petersen RC, et al. 1999. Postmenopausal estrogen replacement therapy and risk of AD. Neurology 52:965–70.

White LR, Petrovitch H, Ross GW, et al. 2000. Brain aging and midlife tofu consumption. J Am Coll Nutr 19:242–55.

Wisniewski AB, Nguyen TT, Dobs AS. 2002. Evaluation of high-dose estrogen and high-dose estrogen plus methyltestosterone treatment on cognitive task performance in postmenopausal women. Horm Res 58:150–55.

Wolf OT. 2003. Cognitive functions and sex steroids. Ann Endocrinol (Paris) 64:158–61.

Wolf OT, Kirschbaum C. 2002. Endogenous estradiol and testosterone levels are associated with cognitive performance in older women and men. Horm Behav 41:259–66.

Wolf OT, Kudielka BM, Hellhammer DH, et al. 1999. Two weeks of transdermal estradiol treatment in postmenopausal elderly women and its effect on memory and mood. Psychoneuroendocrinology 24:727–41.

Woo J, Lau E, Ho SC, et al. 2003. Comparison of *Pueraria lobata* with hormone replacement therapy in treating the adverse health consequences of menopause. Menopause 10:352–61.

Wren BG. 1998. Megatrials of hormonal replacement therapy. Drugs Aging 12:343–48.

Wu FC, von Eckardstein A. 2003. Androgens and coronary artery disease. Endocr Rev 24:183–217.

Yaffe K, Grady D, Pressman A, et al. 1998. Serum estrogen levels, cognitive performance, and risk of cognitive decline in older community women. J Am Geriatr Soc 46:816–21.

Yaffe K, Haan M, Byers A, et al. 2000. Estrogen use, ApoE, and cognitive decline. Neurology 54:1949–53.

Yaffe K, Krueger K, Sarkar S, et al. 2001. Cognitive function in postmenopausal women treated with raloxifene. N Engl J Med 344:1207–13.

Yaffe K, Lui L-Y, Grady D, et al. 2000. Cognitive decline in women in relation to non-protein-bound oestradiol concentrations. Lancet 356:708–12.

Yaffe K, Sawaya G, Lieberburg I, et al. 1998. Estrogen therapy in postmenopausal women. JAMA 279:688–95.

Yoon B-K, Kim DK, Kang Y, et al. 2003. Hormone replacement therapy in postmenopausal women with Alzheimer's disease: a randomized, prospective study. Fertil Steril 79:274–80.

Zandi PP, Carlson MC, Plassman BL, et al. 2002. Hormone replacement therapy and incidence of Alzheimer disease in older women: the Cache County Study. JAMA 288:2123–29.

Zhao L, Chen Q, Diaz-Brinton R. 2002. Neuroprotective and neurotrophic efficacy of phytoestrogens in cultured hippocampal neurons. Exp Biol Med 227:509–10.

CHAPTER THREE

Clinical Data from Structural and Functional Brain Imaging on Estrogen's Effects in the Central Nervous System

DANIEL H. S. SILVERMAN, M.D., Ph.D., CHERI L. GEIST, B.A., AND NATALIE L. RASGON, M.D., Ph.D.

Until recently, little was known about the gender-associated effects of gonadal steroids on neuronal function and neurochemistry. Information about the effects of estrogen on the human brain has recently been provided by studies employing positron emission tomography (PET), functional magnetic resonance imaging (fMRI), and structural (conventional) magnetic resonance imaging (MRI). Studies have focused on the effects of estrogen in healthy premenopausal women, in healthy aging of postmenopausal women, and in pathological aging of postmenopausal women.

PET and Healthy Premenopausal Women

PET has been used to directly quantify several processes relevant to the status of cerebral health and function. These processes include cerebral blood flow (CBF), cerebral blood volume, cerebral rate of oxygen metabolism, and cerebral use of glucose. Clinically, the most commonly performed PET studies of the brain are carried out with [18F]fluorodeoxyglucose (FDG) as the imaged radiopharmaceutical.

In the clinical arena, FDG PET scans are typically interpreted qualitatively, by visual analysis. The reader examines the relative distribution of FDG throughout the patient's brain and compares it with the distribution expected

for a normal subject of similar age. The patient's age is relevant, because cerebral metabolism changes in the course of normal development and aging.
Other factors that can influence scans of normal subjects with respect to either
regional activity or overall count rates include sex, handedness, sensory environment, level of alertness, mood, drug effects, serum glucose levels, and
head fraction (the amount of administered tracer that passes into the brain).

Visual analysis is also used in some research studies, but often the results
of semiquantitative or absolute quantitative analyses are reported in addition
to (or instead of) visual interpretation. In this context, *semiquantitative* refers
to results that are based on regional concentrations of measured radioactivity, normalized to some internal reference standard—for example, a reference
region of the brain, the whole-brain activity, or the average whole-body concentration before excretion and decay—corrected to the actual time of imaging
(i.e., standardized uptake value, or SUV). Those results are adequate for most
clinical applications and for many research applications. In contrast, *absolute
quantitative* values are derived from biologically based mathematical models
that reflect the partitioning of radioactivity into compartments that can reflect
both physiological boundaries (e.g., the vascular space, the blood-brain barrier, the plasma membrane of neurons) and biochemical processes (enzymatic
anabolism and degradation, transport molecules). These models, which necessarily represent a substantial simplification of the actual biological environment, nevertheless have proved capable of yielding quantitative estimates
in good agreement with similar measures obtained by more invasive methods.
In the case of FDG studies, the biological parameter that is being estimated is
the rate of regional use of glucose, based on a method described by Sokoloff
and colleagues (1977) that was originally developed with (unfluorinated) ^{14}C-
labeled 2-deoxyglucose. Early measures of regional use of glucose in the human brain (Huang et al., 1980; Kuhl et al., 1980; Mazziotta et al., 1981; Phelps
et al., 1979; Reivich et al., 1979) yielded estimates of global cerebral metabolism of approximately 5.5 mg glucose/min/100 g, with a range of 3.6–5.2 mg
glucose/min/100 g in white matter structures to 5.8–10.3 mg glucose/min/100
g in gray matter structures. The study by Yamaji et al. (2000) is notable for having obtained regional SUV measurements in the same group of subjects in
which absolute quantitative values were obtained, with remarkably close cor-
respondence of the two types of measure seen in healthy brain (Table 3.1).

With the use of FDG PET, Reiman et al. (1996) located specific brain regions that varied in glucose metabolism during different phases of the menstrual cycle. Ten healthy 18- to 29-year-old women were first scanned during

TABLE 3.1
Rates of Regional Use of Glucose Determined with FDG-PET in Normal Subjects

| Region | Regional Use of Glucose (mg/min/100 g) | |
	Yamaji et al., 2000 68 ± 6 y.o. (n = 18)	Standardized Uptake Values
Frontal cortex	7.9	7.7
Sensorimotor strip	8.1	7.8
Parietal cortex	7.8	7.7
Temporal cortex	7.1	7.0
Occipital cortex	7.8	7.7

Source: Silverman and Alavi, 2005, with permission from Elsevier.

the midfollicular phase, when plasma concentrations of estradiol and progesterone were relatively low. They were then scanned during the midluteal phase, when plasma concentrations of estradiol and progesterone were relatively high. Semiquantitative analyses showed no significant difference in whole-brain glucose metabolism between the midluteal and midfollicular phases. Different brain regions were affected during different phases of the normal menstrual cycle. Thalamic, prefrontal, temporoparietal, and inferior temporal regions had significantly higher glucose metabolism during the midfollicular phase (Fig. 3.1A). Superior temporal, anterior temporal, occipital, cerebellar, cingulate, and anterior insular regions had significantly higher glucose metabolism during the midluteal phase (Fig. 3.1B). Brain regions with relatively large fluctuations in glucose metabolism during the menstrual cycle may be pertinent to understanding sex-based differences in brain function, behavior, and behavioral disorders. This study's experimental design limited its statistical power and restricted analysis to the combined effect of estradiol and progesterone. Despite these limitations, it demonstrated the potential of FDG PET to investigate changes during physiological phases of the female hormonal milieu.

PET has also been used to study the effects of gonadal steroid hormones on the central nervous system (CNS) by measuring regional cerebral blood flow (rCBF). In healthy brain, CBF is normally tightly coupled with local metabolic needs of brain tissue through vasoconstrictive-vasodilatory autoregulation of blood supply. Thus, within a vascular territory, measures of CBF and glucose metabolic rate covary nearly linearly. Between different vascular territories, however, different constants of proportionality can obtain. For example, because most of the lateral neocortex is supplied by the middle cerebral artery branch of the carotid circulation, the pattern of distribution of the

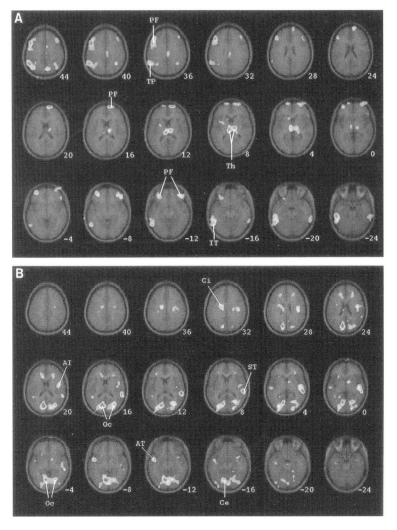

Fig. 3.1 Significant differences in regional glucose metabolism are shown during the midfollicular phase (A) and the midluteal phase (B). Images were constructed using PET and MRI data. The number for each image is the distance in millimeters above (+) or below (−) a horizontal plane between the anterior and posterior commissures. Highlighted areas indicate significance of at least $P < 0.05$.

Source: Reiman et al., 1996: Fig. 2 on p. 2802. © 1996 European Society of Human Reproduction and Embryology. Reproduced by permission of Oxford University Press/Human Reproduction.

blood flow tracer $H_2^{15}O$ closely parallels that of the metabolic tracer FDG throughout most of the cortical surface. Dissociations also occur, however. The cerebellum, despite its lower metabolic activity relative to neocortex, is more richly perfused, being supplied by arterial branches of the vertebrobasilar circulation. Also, in certain pathological circumstances, the normal coupling between metabolism and perfusion can be disturbed, such that a consistent relationship may not exist even within a vascular territory.

Images of regional cerebral activity (rCA) can be obtained with $H_2^{15}O$ (or $^{15}O_2$), as with FDG. In the case of the former tracers, however, the short physical half-life (two minutes) of the ^{15}O nuclide makes them especially suitable for acquiring multiple data sets from the same individual over a relatively brief period. This technique allows for statistical analyses of changes observed in rCA (measured quantitatively or semiquantitatively, as described for FDG) during varying experimental conditions, such as resting versus motor, sensory, or cognitive activities; predrug versus postdrug and withdrawal states; waking versus various stages of sleeping; comfort versus discomfort or pain; and emotional calm versus induced sadness, anxiety, sexual arousal, fear, or anger. This paradigm for studying brain function, known as an activation study, has now been used in thousands of investigations for the purpose of identifying cerebral correlates of normal and pathological processes involved in mentation and behavior.

Fluctuation of gonadal steroid hormones was associated with specific neuronal activity patterns in young, healthy women as assessed by changes in CBF measured with PET. Young, healthy women underwent pharmacologically controlled hormonal conditions (Berman et al., 1997). To induce "menopause," 11 premenopausal women received gonadotropin-releasing hormone (Lupron), followed by either estradiol or progesterone replacement for four to five weeks in a double-blind crossover design. All women performed the Wisconsin Card Sort Test, consisting of working memory, abstract reasoning, and problem-solving tasks. The Wisconsin Card Sort Test physiologically normally activates prefrontal cortical structures, inferior parietal lobule, and posterior temporal gyrus. During the Lupron treatment, patients exhibited altered cerebral activation patterns, but their task performance did not change. Strikingly, the prefrontal cortex in treated women did not exhibit the usual rCBF activation during task performance. The replacement of either estradiol or progesterone restored the activation pattern in the prefrontal cortex (Fig. 3.2). Compared with the progesterone treatment, the estradiol treatment was associated with more activation in the hippocampal area. This PET study showed that the

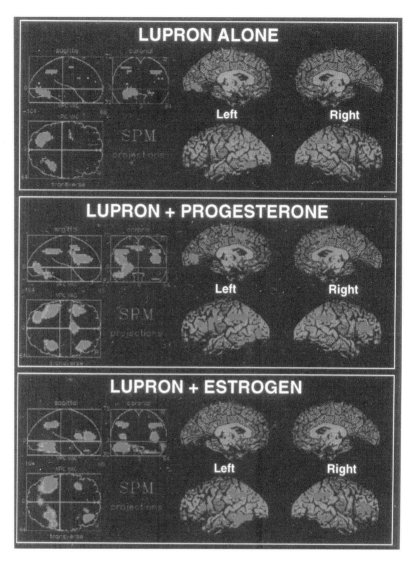

Fig. 3.2 Statistical parametric maps (SPM) show three hormonal conditions. Lighter areas indicate that blood flow during the memory test was greater than activity during the sensorimotor control task.

Source: Berman et al., 1997: Fig. 1 between pp. 8836 and 8841. © 1997 National Academy of Sciences, U.S.A.

hormonal environment could modulate cognitive-related neural activity in women. These results may be interpreted as support for female sex hormones having a facilitative effect on the prefrontal cortex function, which could play a protective role with respect to certain neuropsychiatric illnesses.

fMRI and Healthy Premenopausal Women

The sex-specific effects of blood estrogen levels were examined by Dietrich et al. (2001) in an fMRI study. This noninvasive neuroimaging technique detects differences in the magnetic properties of oxygenated blood, with deoxygenated blood serving as a measure of blood flow. During memory tasks, CBF and oxygen concentration are altered, and these differences can be measured in relative terms for regions associated with the task. Six female and six male subjects underwent fMRI; all subjects completed a word-stem-completion task, a mental rotation task, and a simple motor task. This study found that the healthy female brain is more susceptible than the healthy male brain to changes in cerebral hemodynamics. In addition, the investigators found that the female brain is differently perfused during different phases of the menstrual cycle; peak estrogen levels were associated with an increase in perfusion in cerebral areas involved in cognitive tasks.

PET and Healthy Aging

The effects of normal aging on the brain function of adults have been examined with PET. In a study of 37 healthy adults ranging in age from 19 to 50 years (Schultz et al., 1999), the most significant age-related decline in CBF was found in the mesial frontal cortex, encompassing the anterior cingulate cortex and extending rostrally into the supplementary motor area. In an independent study of 27 healthy adults 19 to 76 years old (Meltzer et al., 2000), the most significant age-related decline was found in the medial orbitofrontal cortex, and this was the only regional effect to remain significant after correction for the partial-volume effects of cerebral atrophy. Measures of metabolism using FDG have also identified an age-related decline in healthy adults (Moeller et al., 1996), most consistently in frontal cortex; nevertheless, as previously reviewed (Mazziotta and Phelps, 1986), studies of carefully selected subjects find declines in glucose metabolism to be minimal throughout most of the brain in normal aging.

MRI and Healthy Aging

Declining levels of estrogen characterize the aging transition from the pre-menopausal to the postmenopausal state, and the transition is often accompanied by changes in brain activation patterns. Numerous estrogen receptors are located in the hippocampus, a region first affected in early Alzheimer disease (AD) (Braak and Braak, 1991). Given the potentially beneficial effect of estrogen in preventing hippocampal atrophy, Den Heijer et al. (2003) used MRI to assess the association between estradiol levels and hippocampal volumes in older men and women. The results indicated that women with higher estradiol levels had smaller hippocampal volumes and poorer memory performance. In men, there was no association between estradiol levels and hippocampal volumes; however, increased estradiol levels were also associated with poorer memory performance. Although the results did not support a beneficial effect of estrogen on the hippocampus and even pointed to an opposite effect, the study suffered from important limitations. There were missing data, and the study tested blood drawn several years before the MRI and memory performance evaluation.

fMRI and Hormone Replacement Therapy in Postmenopausal Women

Older populations are particularly affected by age-associated declines in cognitive function. Using fMRI, Shaywitz et al. (1999) studied brain activation patterns in healthy postmenopausal women before and after a short course of hormone therapy (HT). Women were scanned during performance of verbal and nonverbal working memory tasks in a randomized, double-blind experimental design. Forty-six women underwent two treatments, in random order, for 21 days each: placebo and conjugated estrogens (1.25 mg/day). Statistical analysis revealed that estrogen did not affect memory performance. In contrast, brain activation patterns were significantly affected. Estrogen increased activation in the inferior parietal lobe and superior frontal gyrus during the verbal storage tasks (see Fig. 3.2). These results suggest that the effects of estrogen could be regulated by its action on neural sites controlling phonologically coded information. Furthermore, there was a hemispheric asymmetry effect for both verbal and nonverbal tests (Fig. 3.3). During encod-

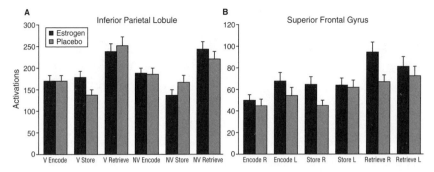

Fig. 3.3 The effects of estrogen in the inferior parietal lobe and superior frontal gyrus. There was a significant increase with the use of estrogen during the verbal (V) tasks (*P* < 0.025) and decrease during the nonverbal (NV) tasks (A). Hemispheric asymmetries are observed (R = right hemisphere, L = left hemisphere) (B).
Source: Shaywitz et al., 1999: Fig. 4 on p. 1200. © 1999 American Medical Association. All rights reserved.

ing, the left hemisphere showed more activation than the right hemisphere. During retrieval, the right hemisphere showed greater activation than the left hemisphere. These findings suggest that estrogen may alter the functional plasticity of memory systems in postmenopausal women without affecting overall cognitive performance.

Volumetric MRI and Estrogen Therapy in Postmenopausal Women

MRI anatomical studies have investigated the effects of estrogen on postmenopausal women. Because of the varied results, researchers hold different views. The differences could reflect differences in experimental design, the statistical tests used, participant age, the healthy-user bias, and the length or type of HT. In a population-based study of older women, Luoto et al. (2000) found that estrogen therapy (ET) users had more clinically significant atrophy than nonusers. In comparisons of past users or nonusers with current users, the bifrontal distance and the size of the ventricles were larger among current ET users. Central measures of atrophy, bifrontal distance, and ventricular size were significantly correlated with cognition as measured by the Mini-Mental State Exam. The results indicated that there is a loss of functioning cerebral tissue related to cognitive decline.

In contrast, Schmidt et al. (1996) found that ET users had less clinically significant atrophy. The MRI study evaluated 70 current ET users and 140 nonusers. The duration and dosage of estrogen replacement regimens varied among users. ET users were better educated and scored significantly better on conceptualization, attention, and visuospatial skills. MRI scans showed that ET users had a lower rate and extent of white matter hyperintensities. The data can be interpreted as indicating that ET users having less silent ischemic brain damage; there was an association among ET, enhanced cognitive functioning, and a reduced rate of ischemic brain damage. Because white matter damage is a predecessor of subcortical arteriosclerotic encephalopathy, it may eventually contribute to the emergence of a dementia syndrome.

Other studies have used MRI to investigate estrogen as a potential neuroprotective agent for healthy postmenopausal women. Eberling et al. (2003) examined gender differences in hippocampal volumes and the effect of ET on age-related hippocampal atrophy in women. Fifty-nine women and 38 men underwent MR, and hippocampal volume was normalized to intracranial volume. The investigators identified no significant effects of gender on normalized hippocampal volumes. Women taking ET had larger right hippocampal volumes than women not taking ET, however, and ET users also had larger anterior hippocampal volumes than men and women not taking ET. Such evidence further supports an effect of estrogen on brain structure.

PET and Pathological Aging in Postmenopausal Women

A PET study found an estrogen depletion effect on cerebral glucose metabolism in older women (Eberling et al., 2000). The study was designed with three different treatment groups: ET users, nonusers, and women with AD. Nonusers did not have any cognitive impairment. Compared with ET users, the AD group had significantly lower regional glucose metabolism. Metabolic ratios for nonusers were intermediate between ratios for users and ratios for the AD group. Cerebral glucose metabolic differences occurred in association with estrogen use for women without cognitive impairment.

A longitudinal study also using PET was conducted by Maki and Resnick (2000). Over a span of two years, they investigated the effects of ET on CBF and cognition in women aged 55 and older. Fifteen ET users and 17 nonusers were scanned under three different conditions: rest, verbal memory task, and figural memory task. When the two patients groups were compared, rCBF in hippocampus, parahippocampal gyrus, and middle temporal lobes was significantly higher in ET users than in nonusers. These regions are part of a memory circuit and are sensitive to preclinical AD. Nonusers had a greater increase in relative pontine CBF. When the neuropsychological performance of the two patient groups was compared, ET users had higher memory scores. As a final point of comparison, the longitudinal effect among ET users revealed a relative increase in hippocampal CBF. These results suggest that ET regulates longitudinal changes in the CBF of regions implicated in AD. These findings also suggest a possible mechanism through which ET could protect against the risk of AD. In a meta-analysis of ET studies, Hogervorst et al. (2000) pointed out that many epidemiological studies suggest that ET exhibits a neuroprotective effect against the development of clinically diagnosed AD; however, poor recall of patient ET use and altered physician behavior may have confounded the effects. Prior patient health, medication compliance, ET type, ET dose, duration of ET, patient heterogeneity, and patient mood could not be controlled rigorously in epidemiological studies.

Neuroimaging studies can also be used to assess the effects of estrogen by comparing patients with pathology and postmenopausal patients. A recent study (Geist et al., 2004) examined the relationship between depression and regional brain metabolism in hypothyroid versus hypoestrogenic depressed patients. Twenty-five women were prospectively studied—11 newly diagnosed, untreated hypothyroid patients (44 ± 14 years) with neuropsychiatric symptoms, 8 age-matched controls (41 ± 14 years) without thyroid disease or neuropsychiatric disorders, and 6 hypoestrogenic (postmenopausal, no estrogen therapy) women with depression. All subjects underwent comprehensive neuropsychiatric assessment, thyroid testing, and FDG PET imaging. The severity of depression was quantified with the 28- and 17-question Hamilton Depression Rating Scales. The severity of depression in hypothyroid subjects correlated most closely with the severity of hypometabolism in the inferior frontal cortex among all regions examined; a tendency toward a correlation with metabolic activity in this region was observed for hypoestrogenic women, but in the opposite direction. In the hypoestrogenic group, depression severity correlated best with hypometabolism in the (left) Broca's area (Fig. 3.4) and was uncorrelated with metabolism in its contralateral counterpart. When the metabolism in each region was compared between patient groups, metabolism in the (left) Wernicke's area differed the most significantly, being lower in hypoestrogenic subjects than in hypothyroid subjects. The severity of

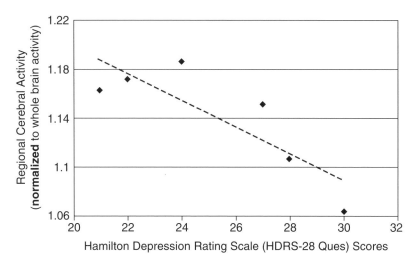

Fig. 3.4 For postmenopausal women, the severity of depression is inversely related to the cerebral activity in the left Broca's area ($r = -0.84$, $P = 0.04$), especially for HDRS scores greater than 24.

depression correlated most closely with hypometabolism in distinct frontal cortical regions in each patient group. On both intergroup comparisons and intragroup correlative analyses, lower metabolism in regions known to be important to language function (Broca's and Wernicke's areas) appeared to be more strongly linked to hypoestrogenism.

In addition to the studies investigating healthy postmenopausal women, neuroimaging has also been used to study the effects of estrogen in unhealthy postmenopausal women. In a PET study, Eberling et al. (2004) examined the effects of estrogen and tamoxifen on brain structure and function. Tamoxifen is a selective estrogen modulator that is given to women with breast cancer. Eberling et al. compared brain glucose metabolism in three groups of postmenopausal women: ET users, nonusers, and women with breast cancer who were taking tamoxifen. When compared with ET users and nonusers, the tamoxifen group showed hypometabolism in inferior and dorsolateral frontal cortex (Fig. 3.5). Compared with ET users, nonusers had decreased metabolism in the inferior frontal cortex and temporal cortex. The tamoxifen group had lower memory scores than the other two groups. Finally, the tamoxifen group had smaller right hippocampal volumes than ET users ($P = 0.05$) (Fig. 3.6). This association was highly significant when an outlier was removed

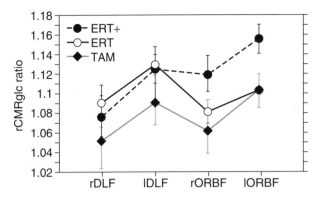

Fig. 3.5 ROI analysis was performed on ERT users (ERT+), nonusers (ERT), and tamoxifen users (TAM). Right and left dorsolateral frontal cortex are represented by rDLF and lDLF, respectively. rORBF and lORBF indicate right and left orbital frontal cortex. *Source:* Eberling et al., 2004: Fig. 3 on p. 367. Reprinted with permission from Elsevier.

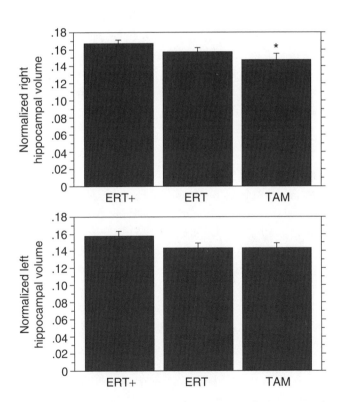

Fig. 3.6 Hippocampal volumes are normalized for women taking estrogen for each group. Standard deviation is shown by error bars. ERT+ indicates women taking ERT therapy; ERT represents nonusers; TAM indicates women taking tamoxifen. *Source:* Eberling et al., 2004: Fig. 4 on p. 367. Reprinted with permission from Elsevier.

($P < 0.05$). These findings would be consistent with estrogen's having a neuroprotective effect. The effects related to tamoxifen in this study are regarded as associations rather than direct effects because they could also have been due to factors associated with having breast cancer.

fMRI and SERMs

Little is known about the effects of selective estrogen receptor modulators (SERMs) on the CNS. Using fMRI, the cerebral effects of the SERM raloxifene were investigated in postmenopausal women during a memory task (Neele et al., 2001). Twenty postmenopausal women were included in the double-blind, placebo-controlled, randomized study. During visual encoding, raloxifene affected brain activation. When raloxifene treatment was compared with placebo treatment, there was a decrease in activation in the left parahippocampal gyrus and left lingual gyrus and an increase in activation in the right superior frontal gyrus. No such effect was observed during recognition and photic stimulation tests. Although additional studies are needed, this study showed that raloxifene may alter brain activation patterns in areas associated with cognitive functioning.

Conclusion

PET, fMRI, and MRI have been used to investigate the cerebral effects of estrogen in normal healthy women, in postmenopausal women aging in a healthy fashion, and in postmenopausal women with pathological aging. Studies of healthy women show that the menstrual cycle can influence neuroimaging measures of brain function. The influence of hormonal levels may also be pertinent to the aging process, which is characterized by estrogen decline. There is increasing evidence that declining estrogen levels may alter cerebral metabolism and the functional plasticity of memory systems in postmenopausal women before affecting overall cognitive performance. In addition, ET may protect brain areas implicated in AD by regulating longitudinal changes in CBF. These early results, although still limited, are encouraging; additional neuroimaging studies may provide further insight into estrogen-related changes in brain function.

REFERENCES

Berman KR, Schmidt PJ, Rubinow DR, et al. 1997. Modulation of cognition-specific cortical activity by gonadal steroids: a positron-emission tomography study in women. Proc Natl Acad Sci USA 94:8836–41.

Braak H, Braak E. 1991. Neuropathological staging of Alzheimer-related changes. Acta Neuropathol 82:239–59.

Den Heijer TD, Geerlings MI, Hofman A, et al. 2003. Higher estrogen levels are not associated with larger hippocampi and better memory performance. Arch Neurol 60:213–20.

Dietrich T, Krings T, Neulen J, et al. 2001. Effects of blood estrogen level on cortical activation patterns during cognitive activation as measured by functional MRI. Neuroimage 13:425–32.

Eberling JL, Reed BR, Coleman JE, et al. 2000. Effect of estrogen on cerebral glucose metabolism in postmenopausal women. Neurology 55:876–77.

Eberling JL, Wu C, Haan MN, et al. 2003. Preliminary evidence that estrogen protects against age-related hippocampal atrophy. Neurobiol Aging 24:725–32.

Eberling JL, Wu C, Tong-Turnbeaugh R, et al. 2004. Estrogen-and tamoxifen-associated effects on brain structure and function. Neuroimage 21:364–71.

Geist CL, Rasgon NL, Bauer MJ, et al. 2004. Regional brain metabolism in depressed women: comparison of hypothyroidism and hypoestrogenism. J Nucl Med 45(Suppl): 67P.

Hogervorst E, Williams J, Budge M, et al. 2000. The nature of the effect of female gonadal hormone replacement therapy on cognitive function in post-menopausal women: a meta-analysis. Neuroscience 101:485–512.

Huang SC, Phelps ME, Hoffman EJ, et al. 1980. Noninvasive determination of local cerebral metabolic rate of glucose in man. Am J Physiol 238:E69–82.

Kuhl DE, Phelps ME, Kowell AP, et al. 1980. Effects of stroke on local cerebral metabolism and perfusion: mapping local metabolism and perfusion in normal and ischemic brain by emission computed tomography of ^{18}FDG and ^{13}NH$_3$. Ann Neurol 8:47–60.

Luoto R, Manolio T, Meilahn E, et al. 2000. Estrogen replacement therapy and MRI-demonstrated cerebral infarcts, white matter changes, and brain atrophy in older women: the Cardiovascular Health Study. J Am Geriatr Soc 48:467–72.

Maki PM, Resnick SM. 2000. Longitudinal effects of estrogen replacement therapy on PET cerebral blood flow and cognition. Neurobiol Aging 21:373–83.

Mazziotta JC, Phelps ME. 1986. Positron emission tomography studies of the brain. In *Positron Emission Tomography and Autoradiography: Principles and Applications for the Brain and Heart,* ed. M Phelps, J Mazziotta, H Schelbert, 493–579. New York: Raven Press.

Mazziotta JC, Phelps ME, Miller J, et al. 1981. Tomographic mapping of human cerebral metabolism: normal unstimulated state. Neurology 31:503–16.

Meltzer CC, Cantwell MN, Greer PJ, et al. 2000. Does cerebral blood flow decline in healthy aging? a PET study with partial-volume correction. J Nucl Med 41:1842–48.

Moeller JR, Ishikawa T, Dhawan V, et al. 1996. The metabolic topography of normal aging. J Cereb Blood Flow Metab 16:385–98.

Neele SJ, Rombouts SA, Bierlaagh MA, et al. 2001. Raloxifene affects brain activation patterns in postmenopausal women during visual encoding. J Clin Endocrinol Metabol 86:1422–24.

Phelps ME, Huang SC, Hoffman EJ, et al. 1979. Tomographic measurement of local cerebral glucose metabolic rate in humans with (F-18)2-fluoro-2-deoxyglucose: validation of method. Ann Neurol 6:371–88.

Reiman EM, Armstrong SM, Matt KS, et al. 1996. The application of positron emission tomography to the study of the normal menstrual cycle. Hum Reprod 11:2799–805.

Reivich M, Kuhl D, Wolf A, et al. 1979. The [18]fluorodeoxyglucose method for the measurement of local cerebral glucose utilization in man. Circ Res 44:127–37.

Schmidt R, Fazekas F, Reinhart B, et al. 1996. Estrogen replacement therapy in older women: a neuropsychological and brain MRI study. J Am Geriatr Soc 44:1307–13.

Schultz SK, O'Leary DS, Boles Ponto LL, et al. 1999. Age-related changes in regional cerebral blood flow among young to mid-life adults. Neuroreport 10:2493–96.

Shaywitz SE, Bennett A, Shaywitz BA, et al. 1999. Effect of estrogen on brain activation patterns in postmenopausal women during working memory tasks. JAMA 281:1197–1202.

Silverman DHS, Alavi A. 2005. PET imaging in the assessment of normal and impaired cognitive function. Radiol Clin North Am 43:67–77.

Sokoloff L, Reivich M, Kennedy C, et al. 1977. The [14C]deoxyglucose method for the measurement of local cerebral glucose utilization: theory, procedure and normal values in the conscious and anesthesized albino rat. J Neurochem 28:897–916.

Yamaji S, Ishii K, Sasaki M, et al. 2000. Evaluation of standardized uptake value to assess cerebral glucose metabolism. Clin Nucl Med 25:11–16.

CHAPTER FOUR

Clinical Data on Estrogen's Effects on Mood

NATALIE L. RASGON, M.D., Ph.D., LAUREL N. ZAPPERT, M.S.,
AND KATHERINE E. WILLIAMS, M.D.

One of the most consistent and intriguing findings in affective disorders research is the increased prevalence of major depression in women. Women are twice as likely as men to have unipolar major depression. Since this increased rate of depression is cross-cultural and appears to begin at puberty and decline after menopause, researchers have questioned the role of gonadal hormones in the different rates of mood disorders between men and women. Estrogen has been postulated to play a role in the regulation of mood since the end of the nineteenth century, when extracts of animal ovarian tissue were administered to oophorectomized women to alleviate psychological symptoms thought to be related to removal of the ovaries (Stoppe and Doren, 2002). Although no correlation between severity of mood symptoms and serum estrogen levels has been consistently found in nonsurgical female populations, the theory that estrogen status affects mood in at least some women is supported by neurobiological studies in animals and humans, and by clinical data obtained across the female human life span. This chapter briefly discusses the biology and neurobiology of estrogen, then reviews the available literature on the use of estrogen, either alone or adjunctively, for the treatment of depression in women.

Theoretical Rationale for the Use of Estrogen in Mood Disorders
Estrogen and Serotonin

A major impetus for investigating the use of estrogens in mood disorders is the clear recognition of the effects of estrogens on multiple areas of serotonergic neurotransmission. Genomic effects of estrogen and estrogen receptors (ERs) on the serotonergic system that have been identified in nonhuman primates include regulation of the rate-limiting catecholamine synthesizing enzyme tryptophan hydroxylase (TPH), which converts tryptophan to 5-hydroxytryptophan (5-HT). In ovariectomized macaque monkeys treated with estrogen or estrogen plus progesterone, there was a ninefold increase in TPH mRNA in the estrogen-treated animals compared with controls. The addition of progesterone increased the TPH mRNA signal fivefold compared with controls (Bethea et al., 2000; Pecins-Thompson et al., 1996). Thus, estrogen alone appears to have the greatest effect on increasing this enzyme, which theoretically leads to increased serotonin synthesis.

Serotonin reuptake is facilitated by the serotonin transporter (SERT); some imaging studies of the serotonin transporter in vivo using positron emission tomography (PET) or single-photon emission computed tomography (SPECT) reported that 5-HT transporter densities are lower in midbrain regions of depressed subjects (reviewed by Staley et al., 1998). A series of experiments in animals and humans suggests that estrogen affects SERT binding. An early method of evaluating SERT binding was through the use of radiolabeled imipramine. Ovariectomized rats treated with estrogen for 12 days demonstrated increased radiolabeled imipramine and serotonin uptake in the frontal cortex and hypothalamus (Rehavi et al., 1987). More selective ligand studies using paroxetine to measure SERT binding sites by autoradiography in ovariectomized rats reported increased binding after estradiol administration in the lateral septum, basolateral amygdala, ventromedial nucleus of the hypothalamus, and ventral nuclei, but not in the periaqueductal gray area, where binding sites were reduced (McQueen et al., 1997). These rat models of SERT binding have an interesting correlate in human studies: in surgically menopausal women, treatment with estrogen led to increased imipramine binding sites on platelets that correlated with improvement in depression scores (Sherwin and Suranyi-Cadotte, 1990).

Estradiol appears to affect 5-HT receptor density in a manner that is region- and time-specific and affected by the presence or absence of progesterone. For instance, in naturally cycling rats, 5-HT1A autoreceptor density is lowest during pre-estrus and estrus, when estrogen levels are highest, and receptor density is highest during diestrus, when estrogen levels are lowest (Biegnon, 1990). Acute administration of estradiol to ovariectomized rats leads to downregulation of 5-HT1A receptors (Osterlund and Hurd, 1998). In ovariectomized monkeys, estrogen treatment and estrogen plus progesterone treatment both led to reduced concentrations of binding sites to 5-HT1A autoreceptors in the dorsal raphe compared to controls (Pecins-Thompson and Bethea, 1998). Thus, since postmortem human studies of depressed subjects have shown that 5-HT1A receptors are increased in the dorsal raphe nucleus, as well as in the hippocampus and cerebral cortex (Stockmeier et al., 1998), the ability of estrogen to modulate these receptors in animal models has lent further theoretical support to the use of estrogen in depressed humans (Osterlund and Hurd, 2001).

Although older, postmortem studies of 5-HT2A receptors in depressed adults demonstrated a changed or increased density of 5-HT2A receptors, in vivo imaging studies have shown contradictory findings, including the observation that long-term treatment with selective serotonin reuptake inhibitors (SSRIs) upregulates these receptors (Staley et al., 1998). The more recent human data accord with animal models of depression and the role of estradiol in the treatment of depression. In rats, 5-HT2A receptor mRNA and protein density decrease after ovariectomy and increase after estradiol administration (Biegnon et al., 1983; Cyr et al., 1998; Sumner and Fink, 1995). Similarly, in an animal model of major depression, the Flinder line sensitive rats, reduced mRNA expression of 5-HT2A receptor in mutant animals was found to be affected by estrogen replacement. Acute treatment with 17β-estradiol led to normalization of 5-HT2A receptor density (Osterlund et al., 1999).

Two recent human studies have shown that estradiol increases 5-HT2A receptor binding in postmenopausal women. Five healthy postmenopausal women who had been free of hormone replacement therapy for at least three months underwent PET at baseline, after 8 to 14 weeks of transdermal 17β-estradiol (1 mg/day), and again after an additional 2 to 6 weeks of transdermal estradiol and micronized progesterone (100 mg twice a day). Treatment with estradiol alone led to significant increases in receptor-binding potential compared with controls in the superior frontal gyrus, ventrolateral prefrontal cortex, inferior parietal lobe, and temporopolar cortex. Administration of combined estrogen plus progesterone was associated with increased receptor binding, with significant changes compared to baseline in the frontal, parietal, temporal, occipital, insular parahippocampal, and posterior cingulate cortices (widespread throughout brain). Estrogen plus progestagen compared with estrogen alone increased receptor binding in medial and lateral orbitofrontal cortex, superior frontal gyrus, parahippocampal gyrus, precuneus, and superior parietal lobe (Moses-Kolko et al., 2003).

In another study, the effects of estrogen on 5-HT2A receptors were correlated with receptor changes and mood in postmenopausal women (Kuyaga et al., 2003). Ten postmenopausal women (at least one year after cessation of menses) with no history of psychiatric illness and free of hormone replacement therapy for at least two months received a transdermal patch of 17β-estradiol (0.075–0.15 mg) for a mean of 10 weeks. Women underwent PET before and after estrogen therapy (ET), and the imaging results were correlated with cognitive assessments, including assessments of verbal memory and executive cognition, and mood assessments, including scores on the Profile of Mood States (POMS) Depression/Dejection subscale and the Beck Depression Inventory (BDI). ET significantly increased 5-HT2A receptor binding primarily in the right prefrontal cortex, but these receptor changes did not correlate with changes on cognitive or mood measures. Increased scores on the Verbal Fluency subscale and improved performance on part A of the Trail Making Test, but not on immediate or delayed paragraph recall or on the Verbal Paired Associates subscale, were seen after treatment. Mood scores were nonsignificantly decreased, but insofar as subjects were already euthymic at baseline, these results were less likely to change. Thus, more studies with larger populations that include symptomatic, depressed patients are needed to further investigate the relationship between estradiol, 5-HT receptor changes, and the treatment of affective disorders.

Estrogen and Norepinephrine

Estrogen has been shown to have effects on the noradrenergic system in both animals and humans. Ovariectomy in rats leads to upregulation of adrenergic receptors in the hypothalamus, corpus callosum, and anterior pituitary (Petrovic et al., 1983), whereas long-term estrogen exposure leads to noradrenergic downregulation (Biegnon et al., 1983) similar to that seen after antidepressant drug treatment in humans. Estrogen also promotes norepinephrine release via a reduction of tonic presynaptic inhibition of α2 autoreceptors (Etgen and Karkanias, 1994).

Estrogen and Brain-Derived Neurotrophic Factor

Brain-derived neurotrophic factor (BDNF) is a nerve growth factor that is believed to have antidepressant effects through its ability to enhance serotonin synthesis (Siuciak et al., 1998) and promote the survival and sprouting of serotonergic fibers (Mamounas et al., 1995, 2000). Increased BDNF leads to increased GABA synthesis and thus increased inhibitory input into pyramidal neurons, while decreased BDNF leads to decreased GABA and increased excitatory cell amplitude. Estradiol appears to affect BDNF mRNA expression in a complex manner that is affected by the duration of the hypoestrogenic state and by acute and chronic estrogen administration. In normally cycling female rats, BDNF mRNA levels were measured and found to be significantly reduced in the hippocampal granular cell layer of the dentate gyrus and the medial prefrontal cortex during pre-estrus, when estrogen levels are highest. In acutely ovariectomized rats, acute administration of estradiol led to a time-dependent decline in hippocampal BDNF mRNA expression, in contrast to chronically ovariectomized rats, in which neither acute nor chronic estrogen affected BDNF expression (Cavus and Duman, 2003). This finding has significant implications for understanding the critical period of efficacy in perimenopause because estradiol may have an important role in early stages, when estrogen levels have just begun to decline, but not as much efficacy in women who have been in menopause for a long time.

The Relationship of Estrogen Changes
to Mood Disorders in Women

From the ample animal data and now the emerging human in vitro and in vivo data, it is evident that estrogen has widespread neurobiological effects on neurotransmitters in brain regions involved in mood regulation. Clinical and experimental studies in humans further suggest that a subgroup of women may be particularly vulnerable to the effects of changing estrogen levels on mood and more likely to respond to estrogen as treatment for depression.

Premenstrual Syndrome and Premenstrual Dysphoric Disorder

Ever since Frank's original description of "premenstrual tension" in the 1930s (Frank, 1931), treatments for premenstrual syndrome (PMS) and premenstrual dysphoric disorder (PMDD) have focused on methods of correcting presumed hormonal "imbalances" that have been implicated in the etiology of the disorder. Early treatments included venipuncture, cathartics, and ovarian irradiation to purge the body of excess estrogen, while later popular treatments focused on adding progesterone supplements to correct a hypothesized progesterone deficiency (Severino and Moline, 1989). Over the past two decades, however, studies have failed to show a difference in mean estrogen or progesterone serum levels across the menstrual cycle between patients with PMS and controls (Dennerstein et al., 1993; Rubinow et al., 1988; Watts et al., 1985).

Researchers have recently reconceptualized the role of estrogen and progesterone in PMS and PMDD. Currently it is proposed that women with severe emotional and physical symptoms have an enhanced sensitivity to either endogenous or exogenous estrogen (Schmidt et al., 1998) or a decreased sensitivity to progesterone metabolites (Rasgon et al., 2001). For instance, women with PMS had more symptoms during menstrual cycles in which luteal phase plasma estrogen levels were highest, including increased breast swelling and tenderness, more irritability, fatigue, and depression (Hammarback et al., 1989). Similarly, women who were randomly assigned to Premarin, 0.625 mg/day, during the luteal phase of the menstrual cycle reported increased mental and physical symptoms of PMS when compared with controls (Dhar and Murphy, 1990).

Although there does not appear to be a role for ET during the luteal phase for PMS, there does appear to be a role for estrogen when it is used all month long in doses high enough to suppress ovulation (Backstrom et al., 1992; Smith et al., 1995). The addition of cylical progesterone analogues to prevent endometrial hyperplasia, however, may be associated with a return of PMS complaints (Watson et al., 1989).

A new oral contraceptive containing estradiol and drospirenone, a spironolactone derivative, has shown promise for the treatment of PMS (Freeman et al., 2001). The most consistently efficacious treatment, however, is with SSRIs (Rapkin et al., 2002).

Postpartum Depression

Postpartum depression affects approximately 10 percent of women. Because it occurs at a time of dramatic hormonal fluctuations, including a rapid decrease in estrogen and progesterone levels, several investigators have attempted to correlate mood with either absolute hormone levels or rate of change. So far, no studies have shown clear differences between estrogen levels in depressed and nondepressed subjects (Hendrick et al., 1998). What has emerged is that women with a history of postpartum depression may have a different sensitivity to changing hormonal levels. For example, in one small study (Bloch et al., 2000), two groups of euthymic women—those with a history of postpartum depression (and no other depressive episodes) and those without—were exposed to the gonadotropin-releasing hormone agonist leuprolide to create a state of hypogonadism, then estrogen and progesterone were added back in supraphysiological doses for eight weeks to simulate the pregnant state. Under double-blind conditions, both estrogen and progesterone were withdrawn. Five of the eight women with a previous history of postpartum depression, but no women in the comparison group, experienced increased depressive symptoms. Although the symptoms were not debilitating, and no women had a score on the Edinburgh Postnatal Depression Scale greater than 10, these women did experience the onset of depressive symptoms. Because the hormonal change was also much less than that experienced during pregnancy and the postpartum period (Bloch et al., 2000), a more dramatic hormonal change would likely be associated with more severe depressive symptoms.

Estrogen Therapy in the Treatment of Postpartum Depression

In an animal model of postpartum depression, female rats were ovariectomized and then stimulated with estrogen and progesterone to simulate pregnancy. In one group of animals hormonal treatment was stopped at the end of the simulated pregnancy; in the other group, estradiol injections were continued. Withdrawal from the gonadal hormones was associated with decreased activity, with more immobility and less swimming on the forced swim test and less struggling, whereas continued estradiol injections appeared to alleviate these depressive symptoms (Galea et al., 2001).

Ahokas et al. (2001) studied 23 women who met criteria for postpartum major depression and measured serum concentrations of 17β-estradiol. They found that levels were low; in fact, in 16 of the 23 patients, estradiol levels were less than 110 pmol/L. Sublingual 17β-estradiol, 1–8 mg/day, was administered for eight weeks and titrated to a serum concentration of 400 pmol/L. The mean dose was 4.8 mg. Cyclical progesterone was added after three months. Treatment response was defined as a 50 percent reduction in the initial depression score. The authors reported that the symptoms improved dramatically in the first week of treatment, with 21 of 23 patients demonstrating treatment response. By the end of week 8, all patients remaining in the study had recovered, defined as a score of less than 7 on the Montgomery-Asberg Depression Rating Scale. The decline in depressive symptoms correlated with a rise in estrogen levels.

In a 1996 study by Gregoire et al., 63 severely depressed women with the onset of depression within three months postpartum received transdermal 17β-estradiol, 200 μg/day, either as monotherapy or as adjunctive therapy to antidepressants. Estradiol was more effective than placebo in treating depression. Because the treatment groups were mixed and no estrogen levels were measured, the findings from this study are difficult to interpret. Thus, both rat and human models of postpartum depression reveal the importance of further examination of estrogen levels in women at high risk for postpartum depression, as well as the possibility that in vivo imaging techniques such as PET may provide further information about serotonin receptor functioning in postpartum depression.

Estrogen in the Perimenopause and Menopause
Definition of Perimenopause and Menopause

Perimenopause is the period of transition from regular menstrual cycles to amenorrhea (Rapkin et al., 2002). During the perimenopausal transition, hormone levels fluctuate erratically as menses become irregular because of intermittent ovulation. The postmenopause is defined by the absence of menstrual bleeding for 12 months and usually occurs between the ages of 45 and 55, with a mean age of 51.4 years (Rapkin et al., 2002). Degeneration of ovarian follicles (apoptosis) occurs, and estrogen levels decline, while pituitary luteinizing hormone (LH) and follicle-stimulating hormone (FSH) levels rise (Rapkin et al., 2002; Steiner et al., 2003). Although mean levels of serum estradiol in premenopausal women are approximately 5 to 35 ng/dL (50–350 pg/mL), levels after menopause fall to approximately 1.3 ng/dL (13 pg/mL). In addition, estrone levels fall from approximately 40–110 ng/dL to 3 ng/dL (Judd, 1994).

As a result of these hormonal fluctuations, women may experience either physical and psychological symptoms, or both. Common mood complaints include irritability, depression, and anxiety. The results of several epidemiological studies and clinic-based surveys suggest that a substantial number of perimenopausal women experience a clinically significant depression (Schmidt et al., 1997). Not all women experience these symptoms, however, and recent data suggest that certain factors predispose women to psychiatric complaints during menopause (Steiner et al., 2003). A personal or family history of affective disorders or mental illness, social stress, and impaired health have all been identified as risk factors for menopausal mood disorders (Banger, 2002; Rapkin et al., 2002), as has a history of mood symptoms at other times of hormonal change.

Novaes et al. (1998) explored the association between a history of premenstrual symptoms and mood symptoms during perimenopause. The authors found that women who currently had perimenopausal symptoms had a significant history of premenstrual dysphoria, and nearly one-third of the subjects met the criteria for a depressive disorder. Specifically, women who had experienced premenstrual dysphoria were more likely to present with psychiatric symptoms, especially depression, during menopause.

Research has also shown that a lengthy perimenopause is associated with higher rates of depression (Rapkin et al., 2002). Avis et al. (1994) conducted a longitudinal follow-up analysis of data obtained on 2,565 women who were 45 to 55 years old when they entered the Massachusetts Women's Health Study. Prior depression proved to be the variable that was most predictive of subsequent depression, and the onset of natural menopause was not associated with an increased risk of depression. Women who experienced a long perimenopausal period (at least 27 months), however, were found to have an increased risk for depression. This association between a long perimenopause and depression appeared to be explained by increased menopausal symptoms rather than by the menopause status itself. Additionally, the observed increase in depression during a lengthy perimenopause appeared to be transitory.

The finding that a longer duration of perimenopause increases the risk for depression is further supported by a longitudinal study conducted by Freeman et al. (2004), who evaluated reproductive hormonal levels and menopausal status as predictors of depression in women undergoing the transition to menopause. An increased likelihood of depressive symptoms was found during the transition to menopause and a decreased likelihood was found after menopause, even after adjusting for other predictors of depression, including a history of depression, severe PMS, age, poor sleep, employment status, and race. Individuals with a rapidly increasing FSH profile were less likely to have depressive symptoms, further supporting the concept that a shorter duration of perimenopause is associated with fewer mood symptoms. The likelihood of depressive symptoms also decreased with age compared with premenopausal women. In addition, increasing estradiol levels were significantly associated with depressive symptoms, suggesting that changing hormone levels contribute to dysphoric mood during the transition to menopause and emphasizing the complexity of the interaction between estrogen and mood (Freeman et al., 2004). Thus, just as in animal models, the relationship between mood and behavior is not a simple reflection of low estrogen levels, but rather fluctuating estrogen levels cause changes in mood. The finding that depressive symptoms increased during the transition to menopause and decreased in postmenopausal women emphasizes that certain women are more vulnerable to changing hormone levels.

Alternatively, a history of depression may shorten the duration of a woman's reproductive life. Harlow et al. (2003) investigated the impact of a lifetime history of major depression on an early transition to menopause and found that women with a history of depression had 1.2 times the rate of early perimenopause of women with no history of depression. Specifically, depressed women with more marked depressive symptoms at study enrollment had twice the risk of an earlier premenopausal transition than nondepressed women, and women with greater depressive symptoms who also reported antidepressant use had nearly three times the risk of an earlier perimenopause. Furthermore, women with a lifetime history of depression had lower estradiol levels and higher levels of FSH and LH at study enrollment and follow-up. These results suggest that a lifetime history of major depression may be associated with an early decline in ovarian function.

Estrogen Monotherapy for Affective Disorders in Peri- and Postmenopausal Women

One of the earliest studies on the use of estrogen for treatment-resistant depression in premenopausal and postmenopausal women was performed by Klaiber et al. (1979). Supraphysiological doses of conjugated estrogen (5–25 mg/day, about 5–20 times the usual postmenopausal replacement dose) were administered to 40 female inpatients with a history of severe recurrent major depression unresponsive to all treatments, including electroconvulsive therapy. The estrogen group (n = 23) experienced a mean drop in scores on the Hamilton Depression Rating Scale (HDRS, also known as HAM-D) of 9.2 points, whereas the mean drop in the placebo group (n = 17) was only 0.1 point. Moreover, scores on the HDRS scale dropped 15 points in 6 of the 32 treated women, whereas no one in the placebo group saw a drop of 10 points or more. Age and menopausal status were not significantly related to the amount of improvement obtained. Although some women clearly experienced significant improvement with ET, most of the women treated with estrogen remained highly symptomatic (Klaiber et al., 1979). To the best of our knowledge, this study has not been replicated.

Since Klaiber's original study, several trials have been conducted, with discrepant results. The data have been difficult to interpret because the studies used different estrogen preparations, routes of administration, and dosages. Furthermore, study populations have been varied and have included both perimenopausal and menopausal women, and women with varying intensity and frequency of menopausal physical symptoms. Consequently, meta-analyses have attempted to evaluate these variables and the effects of estrogen on mood. In a review of 111 studies on hormone therapy (HT), Pearce et al. (1995) reported no consistent association between HT and improvement of depression in women who had undergone natural menopause; however, some effects were found for women who had undergone surgical menopause (Miller, 2003). This review covered both experimental and observational studies and found that observational and non-double-blind studies were more likely to report mood improvement with HT, whereas the results of the double-blind studies were more mixed. Whereas only four of seven double-blind studies indicated mood improvement, four of five observational or non-double-blind studies reported mood improvement with HT (Miller, 2003).

A subsequent meta-analysis of 26 studies suggested that HT is effective in reducing menopausal depressed mood (Zweifel and O'Brien, 1997). The overall effect size for HT in this meta-analysis was 0.68, meaning that the average treatment patient had lower levels of depressed mood than 76 percent of the control patients. Analyses of specific HT regimens showed that estrogen alone had a larger effect size than progesterone alone or in combination with estrogen. Interestingly, androgen alone and in combination with estrogen was associated with an even greater reduction in depressed mood. In addition, the effect size was larger among perimenopausal women than among postmenopausal women.

Two double-blind, placebo-controlled studies published in 2000 and 2001, after the meta-analysis by Zweifel and O'Brien was completed, evaluated the efficacy of estrogen as monotherapy for depression. These trials attempted to control for the problems of the previous studies by enrolling a homogeneous perimenopausal population and using the transdermal route of administration of 17β-estradiol. In the study reported by Schmidt et al. (2000), 34 perimenopausal women with either major depressive disorder (MDD) or minor depression received 50 μg of transdermal 17β-estradiol or placebo weekly for the first three weeks, and all received estradiol during weeks 4 through 6. A full or partial therapeutic response was seen in 80 percent of those who received estradiol during the first three weeks, compared with 22 percent of those who received a placebo. Six of seven women with a current diagnosis of MDD and 19 of 24 women with minor depression responded to active treatment. The effects on mood were independent of the presence of hot flushes or sleep disturbance. In fact, for the symptoms of anhedonia and anxiety, a greater improvement occurred in women without hot flushes than in the depressed women with hot flushes. Therefore, if confirmed by studies with larger samples, these findings suggest that HT may have an antidepressant effect independent of its effects on the physical manifestations of perimenopause (Schmidt et al., 2000).

Soares et al. (2001) investigated the efficacy of 100 mg of transdermal 17β-estradiol for the treatment of perimenopausal women with MDD (n = 26), dysthymia (n = 11), or minor depressive disorder (n = 13). Remission was observed in 67 percent of the estradiol group compared to 20 percent in the placebo group ($P < 0.001$). Moreover, scores on the Montgomery-Asberg Depression Rating Scale continued to decrease throughout the 12-week treatment phase, and the antidepressant benefits were sustained over a 4-week washout period. In this study there was no difference in improvement rates between those with MDD, minor depression, or dysthymia (Soares et al., 2001).

Conversely, one post hoc noninterventional study conducted by Canada et al. (2003) investigated differences in affective and somatic depressive complaints in postmenopausal women receiving ET compared with postmenopausal women not receiving ET. The ET group had significantly less severe somatic symptoms than the non-ET group, and affective scores were marginally lower in the ET group than in the non-ET group. Controlling for mood, the authors found that the benefit of ET continued to be significant with respect to somatic symptom levels. Controlling for somatic levels, however, eliminated the effects of ET on affective depression levels. These results suggest that the chief benefit of ET in reducing subsyndromal depression is reflected in the somatic source of depressive complaints.

In an eight-week open-protocol trial, Rasgon et al. (2002) examined the efficacy of ET in 16 perimenopausal women with MDD. Ten antidepressant and ET-naive subjects received oral 17β-estradiol (0.3 mg/day) alone for eight weeks. Six women with treatment-resistant MDD received 17β-estradiol as an adjunct to treatment with fluoxetine. All patients exhibited clinically significant improvement as measured by HDRS scores after the first week of treatment. Of the 10 women who received ET alone, symptoms remitted in six, three partially responded to treatment, and one had not responded by the end of the eight-week treatment period. Of the six women who received estradiol in addition to fluoxetine, symptoms in one patient remitted and five had a partial response. This small, open-label study suggests that for some antidepressant-naive perimenopausal women with MDD, ET may have antidepressant efficacy.

Another open-label study examined the effect of a four-week course of transdermal 17β-estradiol (100 µg/day) on depression in perimenopausal and postmenopausal women (Cohen et al., 2003). Of the 22 women with perimenopausal (n = 10) and postmenopausal (n = 12) depression, 12 met criteria for MDD, 7 for minor depression, and 3 for dysthymia. ET appeared to be most efficacious in the perimenopausal age group, since remission of depression as determined by the MADRS and BDI scales was noted in 6 of the 9 perimenopausal women but in only 2 of the 11 postmenopausal women. This result suggests that depression in perimenopausal women may constitute a distinct reproductive cycle–related mood disturbance that may respond to ET (Cohen et al., 2003). The finding that the length of the hypoestrogenic state may be associated with responsiveness to acute estrogenic treatment is consistent with the animal data previously discussed. The effect of estrogen on the serotonin system in animal models appears to be related in complex ways to length of time since ovariectomy and to acute and extended use of estradiol replacement therapy.

Estrogen Add-On to Treatment for Affective Disorders in Peri- and Postmenopausal Women

Selective serotonin reuptake inhibitors have been particularly helpful for perimenopausal or menopausal women with affective disorders (Altshuler, 2002). Estrogen is thought to augment the effects of traditional antidepressants, such as SSRIs, during the perimenopausal period (Rapkin et al., 2002). Given that estrogen modulates serotonergic function in the central nervous system, it has been proposed that the decreased levels of estrogen associated with menopause may alter the response to serotonergic antidepressants. Halbreich et al. (1995) administered the serotonin agonist meta-chlorophenylpiperazine (m-CPP) to 18 healthy postmenopausal women not taking estrogen replacement therapy and to 15 healthy menstruating women. Compared with the normally menstruating women, the postmenopausal women had a significantly blunted prolactin peak after m-CPP and a somewhat diminished cortisol peak prior to treatment with estrogen. After one month of ET (estraderm, 0.1 mg), cortisol and prolactin responses to m-CPP levels increased significantly (Halbreich et al., 1995).

Not only do these human and animal basic neurobiological studies support the hypothesis that estrogen can augment effects of antidepressants, but clinical studies support this theory as well. Grigoriadis et al. (2003) compared antidepressant response rates and tolerability in younger (<44 years; n = 91) and older women (>50 years; n = 24) who met DSM-IV criteria for MDD with responses in a comparison group of 86 age-matched men. The most significant finding was that the younger women had significantly lower HDRS scores after eight weeks of antidepressant treatment and achieved significantly higher rates of remission than the older women. This pattern was not replicated in the male control group and underscores the role of estrogenic milieu in gender-specific antidepressant treatment response.

This enhanced treatment response with estrogen may be specific to SSRIs. Kornstein et al. (2000) also reported significant differences between pre- and postmenopausal women in the rate of response to sertraline in a large clinical trial of 235 men and 400 women with chronic major depression or "double depression" (major depressive episodes superimposed on dysthymia). In this study, women were significantly more likely to show a favorable response to sertraline than to imipramine, whereas men responded better to imipramine. A comparison of treatment response rates by menopausal status showed that premenopausal women responded significantly better to sertraline than to imipramine and that postmenopausal women had similar rates of response to the two medications. The authors conclude that female sex hormones may enhance responses to SSRIs or inhibit response to tricyclic antidepressants (TCAs) (Kornstein et al., 2000).

Clinical studies of the use of estrogen to augment the effects of TCAs also show this antidepressant specificity response in that estrogen augmentation of TCAs does not appear to be as beneficial as estrogen augmentation of SSRIs. Two early studies that looked at TCA augmentation with estrogen in women of various ages did not show any additional benefit. In one study, conducted by Shapira et al. (1985), 11 women who had been previously unresponsive to antidepressant treatment received estrogen augmentation after two weeks of treatment with imipramine alone. No significant improvement in HDRS scores was seen four weeks after the addition of estrogen. One patient did show a striking improvement after one week of estrogen augmentation, and another subject with bipolar disorder developed florid mania nine days after estrogen introduction. Other authors have also noted the induction of manic symptoms with the addition of estrogen to antidepressant therapy (Oppenheim, 1984; Young et al., 1997).

Consequently, the strategy of adding estrogen to augment the effects of TCAs warrants further study before it can be endorsed as an intervention for the treatment of unresponsive patients. Further studies should evaluate age and estrogen status in women and clarify the length of time in perimenopause, as well as measurement of TCA levels. The strategy of estrogen augmentation in peri- and postmenopausal women with no or partial response to SSRIs is a little more promising. Other than preliminary data, there are no prospective double-blind studies published. In a post hoc analysis of a six-week trial of fluoxetine (20 mg/day), Schneider et al. (1997) found that 20 percent of 358 subjects had been using concurrent HT in various forms and doses. All subjects were over age 60 and had been diagnosed with MDD. Patients taking ET who received fluoxetine had substantially greater improvement in mean HDRS scores than patients taking ET who received placebo (40.1% versus 17.0%, respectively). Among the women not using ET, there was little difference in response between fluoxetine-treated patients and placebo-treated patients (Schneider et al., 1997). However, Amsterdam et al. (1999), in a retrospective study of women 45 years old and older with MDD, did not find any difference in response to fluoxetine (20 mg) in subjects taking HT (n = 40) compared with subjects not taking HT (n = 132). In 2001, Schneider et al. evaluated the data from two multicenter trials that analyzed the effect of adjunct estrogen on response to sertraline in 127 women over 60 years of age. Although there were no significant differences in HDRS or HAM-A scores, women who were taking ET concurrently (without progesterone) had significantly greater global improvement and quality-of-life scores than those taking sertraline alone. In addition, women who were between the ages of 60 and 64 were more likely to show a clinical response to sertraline than older women.

In the study by Rasgon et al. (2002) mentioned earlier, six women with treatment-resistant MDD received 17β-estradiol as an adjunct to treatment with fluoxetine. One patient experienced symptom remission and five had a partial response. The mean HDRS score at entry was 23.20, compared to 10.6 at the end of the eight-week trial. Of note, a rapid decrease in HDRS scores was apparent following the first week of ET treatment. Similar findings were reported by Westlund and Parry (2003) in a study in which five perimenopausal women diagnosed with MDD were randomly assigned to receive sequentially either fluoxetine (10–20 mg alone), an estradiol patch (0.1–0.2 mg alone), or a combination of fluoxetine and estradiol. Each woman served as her own control. The authors noted that all women reported the most significant improvement in depressive symptoms with the combination treatment.

The effects of ET in the acceleration of antidepressant response in a placebo-controlled design were recently evaluated in 22 postmenopausal women with MDD (Rasgon et al., in press). Subjects received sertraline, 50 mg/day for one week, with an increase to 100 mg/day at week 2, for a 10-week trial; transdermal estrogen or placebo patches were randomly administered concurrently with the initiation of sertraline treatment. The HDRS test was administered to all patients at baseline and weekly thereafter, with both groups showing a significant reduction in HDRS scores by the end of the study. However, the women who received sertraline with ET improved significantly more rapidly than the women who received sertraline with placebo. These results suggest that ET may play a role in accelerating the antidepressant response in postmenopausal women with MDD. To our knowledge, no other studies to date have investigated the acceleration of SSRI response in postmenopausal women.

One reason why these estrogen augmentation studies produce different findings is that estrogen appears to affect SSRI levels, just as it has been known to affect TCA levels. Taylor et al. (2004) reported that administration of fluoxetine and estrogen to ovariectomized rats led to decreased estrogen levels. The authors hypothesized that it was due to cytochrome P450 inhibition. Thus, further augmentation studies should measure estrogen levels and explore whether treatment response is related to unique hepatic metabolism profiles of individual subjects.

Conclusions

The results of basic neurobiological and clinical studies in animals and humans support further investigation of the use of estrogen in selected groups of women during times of hormonal change and mood instability, such as the postpartum period and during the perimenopausal transition. During the reproductive years, women are twice as likely as men to have depression. Although there are numerous explanations for this phenomenon, the most important defining variable is the difference in sex hormones and their actions on different neurotransmitters in the central nervous system.

During the menopausal transition, a subset of women vulnerable to changes in estrogen levels may experience either the recurrence or the new onset of mood disorders, with a direct correlation to the length of the transition. Alternatively, women with a history of MDD may enter menopause earlier than women without such a history. There appears to be a reciprocal influence between MDD and length of reproductive life. Estrogen alone may be effective in the short-term treatment of mild MDD, minor depression, or dysthymia in perimenopausal women. There is no evidence that estrogen by itself is effective in the treatment of MDD in older women, although estrogen may be effective as an adjunct to antidepressant therapy, particularly in peri- and postmenopausal women.

Additional studies of longer duration and with better control are needed to define strategies for the use of estrogen in the treatment of depression in women. Of particular interest is identifying women who would be likely to respond well to estrogen monotherapy and augmentation. Studies supported by the Women's Health Initiative indicate it is crucial to define the risks and benefits of ET and to identify the subset of subjects whose mood symptoms appear to be uniquely dependent on estrogen status. At present, the risks and benefits of ET must be carefully balanced before treatment decisions can be made.

REFERENCES

Ahokas A, Kaukoranta J, Wahlbeck K, et al. 2001. Estrogen deficiency in severe postpartum depression: successful treatment with sublingual physiologic 17beta-estradiol: a preliminary study. J Clin Psychiatry 62:322–26.

Altshuler LL. 2002. The use of SSRIs in depressive disorders specific to women. J Clin Psychiatry 63(Suppl 7):3–8.

Amsterdam J, Garcia-Espana F, Fawcett J, et al. 1999. Fluoxetine efficacy in menopausal women with and without estrogen replacement. J Affect Disord 55:11–17.

Avis NE, Brambilla D, McKinlay SM, et al. 1994. A longitudinal analysis of the association between menopause and depression: results from the Massachusetts Women's Health Study. Ann Epidemiol 4:214–20.

Backstrom T, Hansson-Malmstrom Y, Lindhe BA, et al. 1992. Oral contraceptive in premenstrual syndrome: a randomized comparison of triphasic and monophasic preparations. Contraception 46:253–68.

Banger M. 2002. Affective syndrome during perimenopause. Maturitas 41(Suppl 1): S13–18.

Bethea CL, Mirkes SJ, Shively CA, et al. 2000. Steroid regulation of tryptophan hydroxylase protein in the dorsal raphe of macaques. Biol Psychiatry 47:562–76.

Biegnon A. 1990. Effects of steroid hormones on the serotonergic system. In *The Neuropharmacology of Serotonin*, ed. PM Whitaker-Azmida, SJ Peroutka. Ann N Y Acad Sci 600:427–31.

Biegnon A, Reches A, Synder L, et al. 1983. Serotonergic and noradrenergic receptor in the rat brain: modulation by chronic exposure to ovarian hormones. Life Sci 32: 2015–21.

Bloch M, Schmidt PJ, Danaceau M, et al. 2000. Effects of gonadal steroids in women with a history of postpartum depression. Am J Psychiatry 157:924–30.

Canada SA, Hofkamp M, Gall EP, et al. 2003. Estrogen replacement therapy, subsyndromal depression, and orthostatic blood pressure regulation. Behav Med 29:101–6.

Cavus I, Duman RS. 2003. Influence of estradiol, stress, and 5-HT2A agonist treatment on brain-derived neurotrophic factor expression in female rats. Biol Psychiatry 54:59–69.

Cohen LS, Soares CN, Poitras JR, et al. 2003. Short-term use of estradiol for depression in perimenopausal and postmenopausal women: a preliminary report. Am J Psychiatry 160:1519–22.

Cyr M, Bosse R, Di Paolo T. 1998. Gonadal hormones modulate 5HT2A receptors: emphasis on the rat frontal cortex. Neuroscience 83:829–36.

Dennerstein L, Brown JB, Gotts G, et al. 1993. Menstrual cycle hormonal profiles of women with and without premenstrual syndrome. J Psychosom Obstet Gynecol 14:259–68.

Dhar V, Murphy GE. 1990. Double blind randomized crossover trial of luteal phase estrogens (Premarin) in the premenstrual syndrome (PMS). Psychoneuroendocrinology 15:489–93.

Etgen AM, Karkanias GB. 1994. Estrogen regulation of noradrenergic signaling in the hypothalamus. Psychoneuroendocrinology 19:603–10.

Frank RT. 1931. Hormonal causes of premenstrual tension. Arch Neurol Psychiatry 26:1053–57.

Freeman EW, Kroll R, Rapkin A, et al. 2001. Evaluation of a unique oral contraceptive in the treatment of premenstrual dysphoric disorder. J Womens Health Gend Based Med 20:561–96.

Freeman EW, Sammel MD, Liu L, et al. 2004. Hormones and menopausal status as predictors of depression in women in transition to menopause. Arch Gen Psychiatry 61:62–70.

Galea LA, Wide JK, Alasdair MB. 2001. Estradiol alleviates depressive-like symptoms in a novel animal model of post-partum depression. Behav Brain Res 122:1–9.

Gregoire AJP, Kumar R, Everitt B, et al. 1996. Transdermal oestrogen for treatment of severe postnatal depression. Lancet 347:930–33.

Grigoriadis S, Kennedy SH, Bagby RM. 2003. A comparison of antidepressant response in younger and older women. J Clin Psychopharmacol 23:405–7.

Halbreich U, Rojansky N, Palter S, et al. 1995. Estrogen augments serotonergic activity in postmenopausal women. Biol Psychiatry 37:434–41.

Hammarback S, Damber JF, Backstrom T. 1989. Relationship between symptom severity and hormone changes in women with premenstrual syndrome. J Clin Endocrinol Metab 68:125–30.

Harlow BL, Wise LA, Otto MW, et al. 2003. Depression and its influence on reproductive endocrine and menstrual cycle markers associated with perimenopause: the Harvard Study of Moods and Cycles. Arch Gen Psychiatry 60:29–36.

Hendrick V, Altshuler L, Suri R. 1998. Hormonal changes in the postpartum and implications for postpartum depression. Psychosomatics 39:93–101.

Judd HL. 1994. Transdermal estradiol: a potentially improved method of hormone replacement. J Reprod Med 39:343–52.

Klaiber EL, Broverman DM, Vogel W, et al. 1979. Estrogen therapy for severe persistent depressions in women. Arch Gen Psychiatry 36:550–54.

Kornstein SG, Schatzberg AF, Thase ME, et al. 2000. Gender differences in treatment response to sertraline versus imipramine in chronic depression. Am J Psychiatry 157:1445–52.

Kuyaga A, Epperson N, Zoghbi S, et al. 2003. Increase in prefrontal cortex serotonin 2A receptors following estrogen treatment in postmenopausal women. Am J Psychiatry 160:1522–24.

Mamounas LA, Altar CA, Blue ME, et al. 2000. BDNF promotes the regenerative sprouting, but not survival, of injured serotonergic axons in the adult rat brain. J Neurosci 20:771–82.

Mamounas LA, Blue ME, Siuciak JA, et al. 1995. Brain-derived neurotrophic factor promotes the survival and sprouting of serotonergic axons in rat brains. J Neurosci 15:7929–39.

McQueen JK, Wilson H, Fink G. 1997. Estradiol-17 beta increases serotonin transporter (SERT) mRNA levels and the density of SERT-binding sites in female rat brain. Brain Res Mol Brain Res 45:13–23.

Miller KJ. 2003. The other side of estrogen replacement therapy: outcome study results of mood improvement in estrogen users and nonusers. Curr Psychiatry Rep 5:439–44.

Moses-Kolko EL, Greer PJ, Smith G, et al. 2003. Widespread increases of cortical serotonin type 2A receptor availability after hormone therapy in euthymic postmenopausal women. Fertil Steril 80:554–59.

Novaes C, Almeida OP, de Melo NR. 1998. Mental health among perimenopausal women attending a menopause clinic: possible association with premenstrual syndrome? Climacteric 1:264–70.

Oppenheim G. 1984. A case of rapid mood cycling with estrogen: implications for therapy. J Clin Psychiatry 45:34–35.

Osterlund MK, Hurd YL. 1998. Acute 17β estradiol treatment down-regulates serotonin 5-HT1A receptor mRNA expression in the limbic system of female rats. Mol Brain Res 55:169–72.

Osterlund MK, Hurd YL. 2001. Estrogen receptors in the human forebrain and the relation to neuropsychiatric disorders. Prog Neurobiol 64:251–67.

Osterlund M, Overstreet DH, Hurd YL. 1999. The Flinders sensitive line rats, a genetic model of depression, show abnormal serotonin receptor mRNA expression in the brain that is reversed by 17β estradiol. Brain Res Mol Brain Res 10:158–66.

Pearce J, Hawton K, Blake F. 1995. Psychological and sexual symptoms associated with the menopause and the effects of hormone replacement therapy. Br J Psychiatry 167:163–73.

Pecins-Thompson M, Bethea CL. 1998. Ovarian steroid regulation of 5HT1A auto-receptor messenger ribonucleic acid expression in the dorsal raphe of rhesus macaques. Neuroscience 89:267–77.

Pecins-Thompson M, Brown NA, Kohama SC, et al. 1996. Ovarian steroid regulation of tryptophan hydroxylase mRNA expression in rhesus macaques. J Neurosci 16: 7021–29.

Petrovic SI, McDonald JK, DeCastro G, et al. 1983. Regulation of anterior pituitary and brain beta-adrenergic receptors by ovarian steroids. Life Sci 37:1563–70.

Rapkin AJ, Mikacich JA, Moatakef-Imani B, et al. 2002. The clinical nature and formal diagnosis of premenstrual, postpartum, and perimenopausal affective disorders. Curr Psychiatry Rep 4:419–28.

Rasgon NL, Altshuler LL, Fairbanks LA, et al. 2002. Estrogen replacement therapy in the treatment of major depressive disorder in perimenopausal women. J Clin Psychiatry 63(Suppl 7):45–48.

Rasgon NL, Dunkin J, Fairbanks L, et al. In press. Estrogen and response to sertraline in postmenopausal women with major depressive disorder. Reprod Biol Endocrinol.

Rasgon N, Serra M, Biggio G, et al. 2001. Neuroactive steroid-serotonergic interaction: responses to an intravenous L-tryptophan challenge in women with premenstrual syndrome. Eur J Endocrinol 145:25–33.

Rehavi M, Sepcuti H, Weizman A. 1987. Upregulation of imipramine binding and sero-tonin uptake by estradiol in female rat brain. Brain Res 410:135–39.

Rubinow DR, Hoban MC, Grover GN, et al. 1988. Changes in plasma hormones across the menstrual cycle in patients with menstrually related mood disorder and in con-trol subjects. Am J Obstet Gynecol 158:5–11.

Schmidt PJ, Nieman LK, Danaceau MA, et al. 1998. Differential behavioral effects of gonadal steroids in women with and in those without premenstrual syndrome. N Engl J Med 338:209–16.

Schmidt PJ, Nieman L, Danaceau MA, et al. 2000. Estrogen replacement in peri-menopause-related depression: a preliminary report. Am J Obstet Gynecol 183:414–20.

Schmidt PJ, Roca CA, Bloch M, et al. 1997. The perimenopause and affective disorders. Semin Reprod Endocrinol 15:91–100.

Schneider LS, Small GW, Clary CM. 2001. Estrogen replacement therapy and antide-pressant response to sertraline in older depressed women. Am J Geriatr Psychiatry 9:393–99.

Schneider LS, Small GW, Hamilton SH, et al. 1997. Estrogen replacement and response to fluoxetine in a multicenter geriatric depression trial. Fluoxetine Collaborative Study Group. Am J Geriatr Psychiatry 5:97–106.

Severino SK, Moline ML. 1989. *Premenstrual Syndrome: A Clinician's Guide.* New York: Guilford Press.

Shapira B, Oppenheim G, Zohar J, et al. 1985. Lack of efficacy of estrogen supplementation to imipramine in resistant female depressives. Biol Psychiatry 20:576–79.

Sherwin BB, Suranyi-Cadotte BE. 1990. Up-regulatory effect of estrogen on platelet ^{3}H-imipramine binding sites in surgically menopausal women. Biol Psychiatry 28: 339–48.

Siuciak JA, Clark MS, Rind HB, et al. 1998. BDNF induction of tryptophan hydroxylase mRNA levels in the rat brain. J Neurosci Res 52:149–58.

Smith RN, Studd JW, Zamblera D, et al. 1995. A randomized comparison over 8 months of 100 micrograms and 200 micrograms twice weekly doses of transdermal oestradiol in the treatment of severe premenstrual syndrome. Br J Obstet Gynaecol 102:475–84.

Soares CN, Almeida OP, Joffe H, et al. 2001. Efficacy of estradiol for the treatment of depressive disorders in perimenopausal women: a double-blind, randomized, placebo-controlled trial. Arch Gen Psychiatry 58:529–34.

Staley JK, Malison RT, Innis RD. 1998. Imaging of the serotonergic system: interactions of neuroanatomical and functional abnormalities of depression. Biol Psychiatry 44: 534–49.

Steiner M, Dunn E, Born L. 2003. Hormones and mood: from menarche to menopause and beyond. J Affect Disord 74:67–83.

Stockmeier CA, Shapiro LA, Dilley GE, et al. 1998. Increase in serotonin-1A autoreceptors in the midbrain of suicide victims with major depression: postmortem evidence for decreased serotonin activity. J Neurosci 18:7394–401.

Stoppe G, Doren M. 2002. Critical appraisal of effects of estrogen replacement therapy on symptoms of depressed mood. Arch Women Ment Health 5:39–47.

Sumner BE, Fink G. 1995. Estrogen increases the density of 5HT2A receptors in cerebral cortex and nucleus accumbens in the female rat. J Steroid Biochem Mol Biol 54:15–20.

Taylor GT, Farr S, Klinga K, et al. 2004. Chronic fluoxetine suppresses circulating estrogen and the enhanced spatial learning of estrogen-treated ovariectomized rats. Psychoneuroendocrinology 29:1241–49.

Watson NR, Studd JW, Savvas M, et al. 1989. Treatment of severe premenstrual syndrome with oestradiol patches and cyclical oral norethisterone. Lancet 23:730–32.

Watts JF, Butts WR, Edwards RI, et al. 1985. Hormonal studies in women with premenstrual tension. Br J Obstet Gynaecol 92:247–55.

Westlund TL, Parry BL. 2003. Does estrogen enhance the antidepressant effects of fluoxetine? J Affect Disord 77:87–92.

Young RC, Moline M, Kleyman F. 1997. Hormone replacement therapy and late-life mania. Am J Geriatr Psychiatry 5:179–81.

Zweifel JE, O'Brien WH. 1997. A meta-analysis of the effect of hormone replacement therapy upon depressed mood. Psychoneuroendocrinology 22:189–212 [erratum in Psychoneuroendocrinology 22:655, 1997].

CHAPTER FIVE

Preclinical Efforts to Develop Effective NeuroSERMs for the Brain

ROBERTA DIAZ BRINTON, Ph.D., AND LIQIN ZHAO, Ph.D.

Why Focus on Therapeutic Strategies to Prevent Alzheimer Disease?

Neurodegenerative diseases are among the most devastating and costly age-associated maladies. Of the neurodegenerative diseases, Alzheimer disease (AD) is the leading cause of dementia, loss of independent living, and institutionalization (Brookmeyer et al., 1998; Fillit, 2000, 2002a; Whitehouse, 1997). AD can have a prolonged gestational period until frank symptoms develop (up to 20 years), followed by an equally slow rate of debilitation over a period lasting from 1 to 15 years (Fillit et al., 2002).

Age remains the greatest risk factor for developing AD, which typically presents in the mid-seventies and becomes most prevalent in the mid-eighties, with nearly 50 percent of octogenarians manifesting evidence of the disease. Conservative projections indicate that the prevalence of AD will nearly quadruple in the next 50 years, by which time one in 45 Americans will be afflicted with the disease (Brookmeyer et al., 1998). Currently, approximately 360,000 new cases of AD occur each year. To put these numbers into perspective, it is interesting to contrast the incidence of AD and that of AIDS. In the United States, 44,232 new cases of AIDS were reported to the U.S. Centers for Disease Control in 2003, compared with 360,000 new cases of AD (Centers for Disease Control, 2005). In the current therapeutic environment the number of new AD cases is projected to rise more than threefold, from

360,000 new cases per year in 1997 to 1.14 million new cases per year in 2047. In the United States alone, the cost of caring for the 4 million persons who currently have AD is approximately $100 billion per year (Fillit, 2000, 2002a). By 2050, if the rates do not change and if no effective preventive therapies are developed, 14 million older Americans are expected to have AD (Fillit, 2000, 2002a).

Gender Demographics of AD: A Women's Health Issue

Despite high-profile cases such as those of Ronald Reagan, Charlton Heston, and Sargent Shriver, women are by far the principal victims of AD (Brinton, 1999; Fillit, 2002b). Of those affected by AD, 68 percent are female and 32 percent are male (Brookmeyer et al., 1998). Because women have a longer life expectancy than men, the number of women with AD exceeds the number of men. Moreover, a double danger exists for women: the results of a meta-analysis of seven sex-specific studies concluded that women are 1.5 times more likely to develop AD than age-matched men (Gao et al., 1998), a conclusion supported by the Cache County cohort analysis, which showed a clear female gender increase in the incidence of AD (Zandi, Carlson, et al., 2002).

At the turn of the twenty-first century, there were nearly 42 million women over the age of 50 in the United States, and of these, more than 31 million were over the age of 55 (North American Menopause Society, 2003). In the United States, 50 million women are expected to be 55 or older by the year 2020. Currently, a woman's average life expectancy is estimated to be 79.7 years. A woman who reaches the age of 54, however, can expect to live to 84, and nearly two-thirds of the total U.S. population will survive to age 85 or older. Based on these data, women can anticipate spending one-third to one-half of their lifetime in the postmenopausal state. Current epidemiological data indicate that of the 18 million American women now in their seventies and eighties, almost half will manifest the histopathological changes of AD (Henderson, 2000a). Worldwide, more than 470 million women are 50 years old or older, and 30 percent of those are projected to live into their eighties (North American Menopause Society, 2003). The potential impact of AD on society as a whole is overwhelming, because the disease affects both sexes. The projected exponential increase in the prevalence of AD, along with the anticipated impact on families and society, highlights the importance of developing strategies to prevent AD.

Estrogen's Mechanisms of Action in Neurons: Understanding the Clinical Results of Estrogen and Hormone Therapy and AD

By understanding the mechanisms of action of estrogen and progestin in brain, one can predict the efficacy of estrogen therapy (ET) and hormone therapy (HT) in promoting neurological function and preventing neurodegenerative disease (Brinton, 2004a, 2004b; Brinton and Nilsen, 2003; Nilsen and Brinton, 2003a; Nilsen et al., 2002; Zandi, Carlson, et al., 2002). Together, basic science analyses, epidemiological studies, and clinical trial results indicate that the benefits of estrogen action depend on the initial health status of the neurons. If neurons are healthy at the time of exposure to estrogen, their response to estrogen is beneficial for both neuronal function and survival (Figs. 5.1 and 5.2). In contrast, if the neuron is diseased or dysfunctional at the

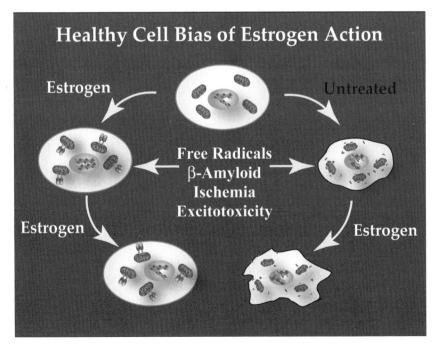

Fig. 5.1 Exposure to estrogen before exposure to neurodegenerative insults induces a proactive defense state, whereas exposure of neurons to estrogen following the insult promotes their demise.

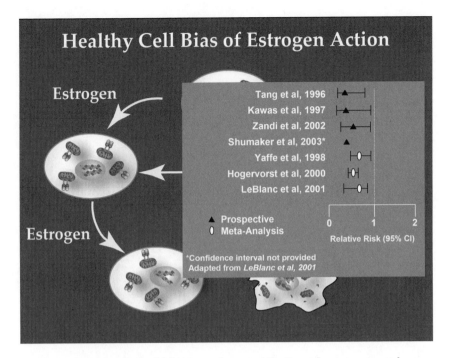

Fig. 5.2 In women treated with hormone therapy at the time of menopause, and presumably before neurodegenerative insults have developed, estrogen therapy reduces the risk of Alzheimer disease.

time of exposure, the effect of estrogen is deleterious (Fig. 5.3). The healthy-cell bias of estrogen action is consistent with epidemiological data indicating a reduction in risk for AD in women who begin ET or HT at the time of menopause, and by the treatment and Women's Health Initiative Memory Study (WHIMS) trials in which women began taking ET or HT either after the disease had developed or decades after menopause (Espeland et al., 2004; Henderson, 2000b; Henderson et al., 2000; Mulnard et al., 2000; Shumaker et al., 2003, 2004; Zandi, Carlson, et al., 2002) (see Fig. 5.3).

Estrogen Activates Calcium Signaling in Neurons: Implications for Neuroprotection, Memory, and Neurodegeneration

In hippocampal neurons, 17β-estradiol (E_2) and other estrogenic ligands bind to an as yet uncharacterized, membrane-associated estrogen receptor

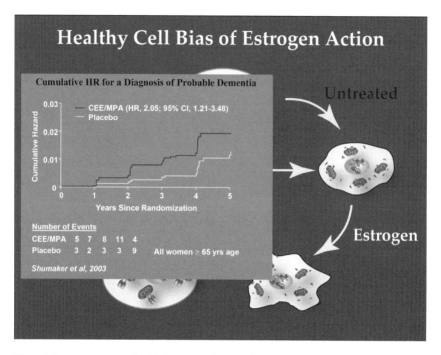

Fig. 5.3 In women treated with hormone therapy decades after menopause, when neurodegenerative insults could have developed, estrogen therapy increases the risk of Alzheimer disease.

(ER) (Kuroki et al., 2000; Razandi et al., 1999; Watson et al., 2002) (Fig. 5.4). The estrogen-bound receptor complex can, in select cell types, bind to and activate the phosphatidylinositol-3-kinase (PI3K) (Simoncini et al., 2000), which in turn activates calcium (Ca^{2+})-independent PKC (Wymann and Pirola, 1998), very likely PKCδ (Lee and Brinton, 2003). We propose that a Ca^{2+}-independent PKC isoform phosphorylates the L-type Ca^{2+} channel, followed by Ca^{2+} influx (Wu et al., 2003). The intracellular Ca^{2+} rise activates conventional Ca^{2+}-dependent PKCs (Cordey et al., 2003), which then phosphorylate and activate Src kinase (Guo et al., 2004; Thomas and Brugge, 1997). Src then activates the MEK/ERK1/2 pathway (Migliaccio et al., 1996; Nethrapalli et al., 2001), which is followed by translocation of activated ERK into the nucleus (Nilsen and Brinton, 2003b; Singh et al., 1999). Activated ERK phosphorylates cAMP response element-binding protein (CREB), which, when activated, can increase transcription of the morphogenesis-related gene spinophilin (Zhao et al., 2005) and the antiapoptotic genes *Bcl-2* (Nilsen and

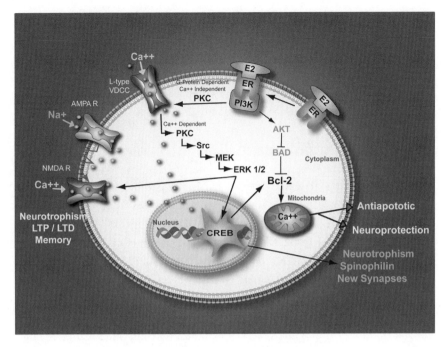

Fig. 5.4 Schematic of estrogen-activated signaling cascade in hippocampal neurons.

Brinton, 2003b) and *Bcl-xl* (Pike, 1999). Subsequent to the activation of CREB, the Src/ERK signaling cascade leads to potentiation of glutamate-dependent activation of α-amino-3-hydroxy-5-methyl-4-isoxazolepropionic acid (AMPA) and N-methyl-D-aspartate (NMDA) receptors (Foy et al., 1999; Nilsen et al., 2002). Activation of both L-type Ca^{2+} and NMDA channels is required for E_2-enhanced long-term potentiation (LTP) and morphogenesis (Bi et al., 2000; Woolley and McEwen, 1994; Zhao et al., 2005). E_2-activated CREB is also re-quired for E_2 induction of spinophilin expression and new synapse forma-tion (Lee et al., 2004; Zhao et al., 2005). In parallel, PI3K also activates Akt (Singh, 2001; Znamensky et al., 2003), which can phosphorylate the proapop-totic protein BAD, preventing heterodimerization with, and inactivation of, *Bcl-2* (Datta et al., 1997). Estrogen, by an as yet unknown mechanism, in-creases mitochondrial sequestration of Ca^{2+}, protecting neurons against the adverse consequences of excess cytoplasmic Ca^{2+} and subsequent dysregula-tion of Ca^{2+} homeostasis (Brinton et al., 2002; Nilsen and Brinton, 2003a). Despite an increased mitochondrial Ca^{2+} load, E_2 promotes mitochondrial function, preserving mitochondrial respiration (Masri et al., 2004; Nilsen and

Brinton, 2004). E_2 could preserve mitochondrial respiration in part through its ability to increase both cytochrome C oxidase protein levels and enzyme activity (Masri et al., 2004). Collectively, the complex signaling cascade activated by E_2 in healthy neurons enhances the biochemical, genomic, and morphological mechanisms of memory, and also proactively induces mechanisms of protection against neurodegenerative insult.

Estrogen Receptors in Hippocampus and Cortex

Two nuclear receptors for estrogen have been identified, ERα and ERβ. Both ERα and ERβ are expressed in hippocampus and cortex from rodent and human brain (Audesirk et al., 2003; Couse et al., 1997; Hu et al., 2003; Lu et al., 2003, 2004; McEwen, 2002; Milner et al., 2001; Mitra et al., 2003; Savaskan et al., 2001; Shughrue and Merchenthaler, 2000; Shughrue et al., 2000; Zhao et al., 2004). We have found that both receptors can promote neuron survival in rat hippocampal neurons (Zhao et al., 2004). The ER in brain responsible for the neuroprotective and neurotrophic actions in brain is not yet fully characterized. In hippocampal neurons, 17β-estradiol (E_2) and other estrogenic ligands bind to a membrane-associated ER (mER) (Brinton, 2001) (see Fig. 5.4). Whether these effects are mediated by nuclear ERs or by mERs is unresolved. The case for a membrane-localized ER in neurons is now well supported by data from multiple laboratories, including our own (Adams et al., 2002; Brinton, 1993, 2001; Brinton et al., 1997; Dubal and Wise, 2001; Dubal et al., 2001; Foy et al., 1999, 2001; Kim et al., 2002; McEwen, 2002; Milner et al., 2001; Mitra et al., 2003; Nilsen and Brinton, 2003a; Shughrue et al., 2000; Simoncini et al., 2000; Singer et al., 1999; Singh et al., 1999, 2001; Toran-Allerand, 2004; Waters et al., 2001; Watson et al., 1995, 2002; Watters et al., 1997; Wu et al., 2005; Zhao et al., 2005). The exact structure and characteristics of the mER, however, remain unresolved. The antigenic properties of hippocampal and cortical mERs exhibit multiple epitope features, as do the nuclear ERs (ERα/β), suggesting that mERs share at least some features in common with nuclear ERs, which points to a common genetic origin.

Window of Opportunity for Estrogen-Induced Benefit

Calcium dynamics play a pivotal and obligatory role in the E_2-inducible cascade that leads to the neurotrophic and neuroprotective benefit of E_2. The dynamics of Ca^{2+} homeostasis are tightly regulated in healthy neurons and dysfunctional in degenerating neurons (Clodfelter et al., 2002; Foster, 2002; Foster and Kumar, 2002; Foster et al., 2003; LaFerla, 2002; LaFerla et al., 1995; Landfield, 1994; Landfield et al., 1992; Leissring et al., 1999; Mattson et al., 2000; Porter and Landfield, 1998; Porter et al., 1997; Thibault and Landfield, 1996; Thibault et al., 1998, 2001). Therein lies the Achilles heel of estrogen action: increasing Ca^{2+} influx into (and sequestration in) cytoplasmic and mitochondrial compartments of neurons unable to maintain Ca^{2+} homeostasis leads to exacerbation of Ca^{2+}-dependent degenerative insults (LaFerla, 2002; Landfield et al., 1992; Mattson et al., 1993; Thibault et al., 1998).

To pursue this hypothesis, we have begun to develop in vitro models simulating prevention versus treatment modes of E_2 exposure. The results of those analyses indicate that hippocampal neurons exposed to E_2 in a prevention model exhibit significantly greater survival than neurons treated with E_2 at the time of β-amyloid insult. In stark contrast, hippocampal neurons exposed to E_2 *after* β-amyloid insult, a treatment paradigm, exhibit less survival than those neurons exposed to β-amyloid alone (Fig. 5.5). These in vitro data are remarkably consistent with epidemiological analyses indicating that women who receive ET preventatively at the time of menopause, well before age-associated degeneration is rampant, have a lower risk of developing AD than women who never receive ET or HT (Carlson et al., 2001; Fillit, 2002b; Henderson, 1997; Henderson et al., 2000; Kawas et al., 1997; Miller et al., 2001; Tang et al., 1996; Yaffe et al., 1998; Zandi, Anthony, et al., 2002). The results from our in vitro "treatment" paradigm are also remarkably consistent with the clinical data indicating that in women who begin HT after the onset of AD or in their sixties or seventies, when age-associated insults have already occurred in some women, ET and HT exacerbate the degenerative state (Espeland et al., 2004; Henderson et al., 2000; Mulnard et al., 2000; Shumaker et al., 2003, 2004; Zandi, Anthony, et al., 2002).

Clinical Implications

The mechanisms of estrogen's action in hippocampal and cortical neurons predict that the use of ET in healthy neurons would result in neurons that were able to defend against neurodegenerative insults such as those associated with AD. In contrast, if neurons are already in a state of degeneration, exposure to ET is likely to exacerbate the degeneration because of the inability of these neurons to effectively regulate the increased calcium load within the cell and within their mitochondria.

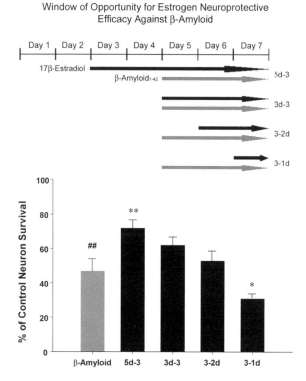

Fig. 5.5 In vitro model for testing "prevention versus treatment" efficacy of E_2 against β-amyloid-induced neuron death.

The Effects of Progestogen on Estrogen-Inducible Responses in the Brain

Our studies indicate that progestins differ dramatically in their effects on neuronal responses and their interaction with estrogen (Brinton and Nilsen, 2003). Specifically, in hippocampal neurons, 17β-estradiol (E_2), progesterone, and 19-norprogesterone, alone or in combination with E_2, are neuroprotective against insults associated with AD and increase the expression of the antiapoptotic protein Bcl-2 (Nilsen and Brinton, 2002b, 2003a, 2004). In striking contrast, medroxyprogesterone acetate (MPA, contained in PremPro) was not neuroprotective, nor did it induce Bcl-2 expression. Moreover, MPA completely antagonized E_2-induced neuroprotection and Bcl-2 expression (Nilsen and Brinton, 2003b). We also found that MPA blocked E_2-inducible memory mechanisms, whereas progesterone exerted a mixed agonist/antagonist effect (Nilsen and Brinton, 2002a). Although the mechanisms underlying the disparity between progestins remain to be fully determined, translocation of signaling molecules (ERK1/2) to the nucleus appears to be crucial and is predictive of neuroprotective efficacy (Nilsen and Brinton, 2003b). E_2 and progesterone, alone or in combination, translocate the mitogen-activated protein kinase (MAPK) extracellular signal–regulated kinase (ERK) to the nucleus, whereas MPA does not, and MPA blocked E_2-induced translocation of ERK (Nilsen and Brinton, 2003b). These studies, conducted while WHIMS was in progress, provide a cellular profile against which current clinical progestins and those in development can be tested for their impact on estrogen-inducible effects in neurons. The results of these analyses could then be used to predict the efficacy of HT formulations for the prevention of AD. Blockade of estrogen-inducible mechanisms of neuroprotection and cognition would be expected to obstruct estrogen protection against insults that culminate in AD, thereby increasing the risk for the disease. The challenge remains to develop a therapeutic strategy for promoting the beneficial effects of estrogen in the brain while preventing the untoward consequences of the hormone in other organ systems.

Clinical Implications

The results of our in vitro studies and of the HT (PremPro) arm of WHIMS indicate that MPA effectively antagonizes estrogen's action in the brain and may even have adverse effects. Our analysis of clinically relevant progestogens indicates that progesterone and 19-norprogesterone synergize with estrogen to increase the proactive defense mechanisms in neurons while only partially antagonizing estrogen activation of memory mechanisms.

How Do We Reap the Benefits of ET or HT for the Prevention of AD Without Encountering the Harm?

One strategy for reaping the benefit of estrogen's preventive effect while safeguarding against harm is simply to administer ET or HT at the time of menopause, and to refrain from administering these therapies years to decades after the menopausal transition (Brinton, 2004a) (Fig. 5.6). The timing of ET is not the only hurdle, however. Only 25 percent of eligible postmenopausal women elect to receive prescribed ET or HT (Hammond, 1994). Of that 25 percent, only 20 percent are compliant with a course of prescribed ET or HT three

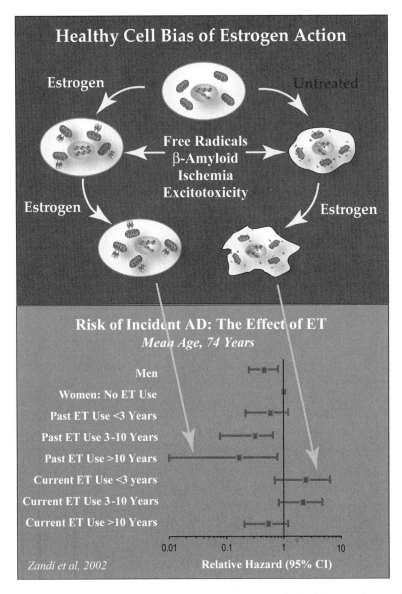

Fig. 5.6 Mechanisms of estrogen action predict a reduced risk of Alzheimer disease if estrogen therapy is initiated before the development of age-related degeneration and an increased risk of Alzheimer disease if estrogen therapy is initiated after age-related degeneration has begun.

years later (Hammond, 1994). The principal reason women forgo ET or HT is the fear of developing breast cancer (Hammond, 1994). In addition, the WHI study that found an increased risk for ischemic stroke (Shumaker et al., 2003) and overall coronary heart disease (CHD) (Manson et al., 2003) in women taking HT or ET has further heightened the fear of adverse effects from ET and HT. Women have indicated that the perceived risks associated with current ET or HT regimens outweigh the perceived benefits.

As an alternative to ET or HT, it may be possible to develop molecules that selectively activate the neuroprotective and memory mechanisms of estrogen in the brain while not activating mechanisms in other tissues that lead to an increased risk of thrombosis and neoplasms. An increasing number of ER ligands and novel selective ER modulators (SERMs) have been identified in nature, while others have been designed and synthesized de novo by academic research institutions and the pharmaceutical industry (Chen, Dykstra, et al., 2004; Chen, Kim, et al., 2004; Gust et al., 2002; Jordan, 2003a, 2003b; Kamada et al., 2004; Katzenellenbogen et al., 2001; Miller, 2002; C.P. Miller et al., 2001; Renaud et al., 2003; Watanabe et al., 2003; C. Yang et al., 2004). The Food and Drug Administration has approved the use of ET and HT for the treatment of hot flushes and the prevention of osteoporosis. Thus, pharmaceutical industry efforts focus on these two endpoints, along with antineoplastic action in breast and uterus. The molecules under development are diverse but have in common that they do not specifically target estrogenic actions in the brain, in particular the actions of mERs.

Our scientific endeavors over the past two decades have focused on determining the neuronal mechanisms of action responsible for promoting estrogen-dependent memory function and neuron survival (Brinton, 2001, 2002; Brinton and Nilsen, 2001; Brinton et al., 1997; Nilsen and Brinton, 2003a; Nilsen et al., 2002; Zhao et al., 2005). These endeavors, together with those of our colleagues in the field, have yielded insights into the mechanisms of estrogen's action that allow us to translate our basic science understanding into the therapeutic design of a brain-selective estrogen, or NeuroSERM (Dykens et al., 2003; Green et al., 1997, 2001; McEwen, 2002; Shi et al., 2001; Simoncini et al., 2000; Singer et al., 1998; Singh, 2001; Singh et al., 1994, 1999, 2000; Watson et al., 1995; Wise et al., 2001; Woolley, 1999; Yang et al., 2004). The goal of our NeuroSERM development efforts is to generate small-molecule therapeutics that can easily penetrate the blood-brain barrier and bind to mERs to activate estrogenic mechanisms that promote cognitive function and prevent age-associated neurodegenerative disease in both women and men (Brinton et al., 2002). The following sections review the results of our analyses of the estrogen agonist action of existing SERMs, followed by a description of our in silico function-driven and structure-based design and development of NeuroSERMs for the prevention of age-related neurodegeneration.

Phytoestrogens

Phytoestrogens are a primary class of plant-derived estrogen alternatives that structurally resemble endogenous estrogen, bind directly to ERs, and regulate gene transcription through estrogen response elements (EREs) (Kurzer and Xu, 1997). Select phytoestrogens have been found to exhibit some estrogen agonist-like properties (Makela et al., 1995; Stahl et al., 1998), but many also act as partial ER antagonists (Bowers et al., 2000). The cellular mechanisms activated by phytoestrogens are diverse and appear to be concentration dependent (Wang and Kurzer, 1997). At low concentrations, phytoestrogens can induce the proliferation of ER-positive MCF-7 cells but not of ER-negative MDA-MB-231 cells (Wang and Kurzer, 1997). Conversely, several studies have shown the antiproliferative effects of phytoestrogens on human breast cancer cell lines and in animal experiments. High concentrations of phytoestrogens (comparable to those achieved in plasma following consistent soy consumption) can significantly inhibit proliferation of human breast carcinoma cell growth (Balabhadrapathruni et al., 2000; Dixon-Shanies and Shaikh, 1999; Wang and Kurzer, 1997; Zava and Duwe, 1997).

To determine whether phytoestrogens exert an estrogen agonist effect in neural tissue, we investigated the neurotrophic and neuroprotective efficacy of six phytoestrogens: genistein, genistin, daidzein, daidzin, formononetin, and equol (Zhao and Brinton, 2002). The results of these analyses indicate that although phytoestrogens exert a modest neuroprotective effect at the plasma membrane, they do not sustain neuronal viability, nor do they induce cellular correlates of memory (Zhao and Brinton, 2002). Data derived from these investigations would predict that phytoestrogens could exert modest neuroprotection analogous to that of antioxidants but that these molecules are not functional equivalents to endogenous 17β-estradiol or to estrogen formulations and therefore would be unlikely to reduce the risk of AD or to sustain memory function in postmenopausal women.

The results of studies in humans are consistent with our in vitro data. Rice and colleagues studied Japanese-American women 65 years old or older to determine the impact of soy consumption and cognitive function (Rice et al.,

1995). They found that women using ET who consumed tofu more than three times per week were not protected against cognitive impairment, but women using ET who consumed tofu less than three times per week were less likely to be cognitively impaired than were nonestrogen users. These results suggest that in women already using ET, tofu consumed in large amounts can block the beneficial effects of ET, thereby acting as an estrogen antagonist. Further, the results of two clinical trials reported in *JAMA* indicate that soy isoflavones are not effective in preventing menopause-associated cognitive decline or in controlling hot flushes (Kreijkamp-Kaspers et al., 2004; Tice et al., 2003).

Tamoxifen

Tamoxifen is a triphenylethylene, nonsteroidal mixed ER agonist/antagonist (Coezy et al., 1982; Jordan and Koerner, 1975). The active metabolic product, 4-hydroxy-tamoxifen (OHT), is a minor metabolite of tamoxifen with a short half-life, but it binds to ER with an affinity 20 to 30 times greater than that of tamoxifen and equivalent to that of 17β-estradiol (Bruning, 1992; Eppenberger et al., 1991; Grill and Pollow, 1991; Jordan et al., 1977; Kawamura et al., 1991). Since 1971, tamoxifen has been used to treat breast cancer in postmenopausal women (Cole et al., 1971), and in 1999 it was recommended for use in breast cancer prevention (Gerber and Krause, 1999). Tamoxifen is characterized as a SERM because of its ER antagonist action in breast, uterus (for five years before conversion to ER agonist in a subset of women), and hypothalamus, whereas it exerts agonist functions in bone, liver, and eventually in the uterus in a subset of women (Mitlak and Cohen, 1997; Shang and Brown, 2002).

We sought to determine whether tamoxifen or its higher-affinity active metabolite, OHT, exerted estrogen agonist action in the brain to promote estrogen-induced mechanisms of neuroprotection and morphogenesis. Our analyses indicated that in the absence of 17β-estradiol, tamoxifen and its metabolite, OHT, were modestly neuroprotective but did not promote cellular features and mechanisms of memory formation. In contrast, in the presence of 17β-estradiol, tamoxifen and OHT functioned as ER competitive antagonists (O'Neill and Brinton, 2001, 2002). These data would predict that in postmenopausal women, in the absence of 17β-estradiol, tamoxifen could act as a modest neuroprotective estrogen agonist in the brain, but in premenopausal (ovaries intact) women, tamoxifen would function as an ER antagonist in the brain. However, neither tamoxifen nor its metabolite, OHT, would promote memory function in postmenopausal or premenopausal women, as neither of these molecules activates the mechanisms required for memory formation. A clinical report by Paganini-Hill and Clark supports the predictions of our basic scientific data. Women who had used tamoxifen for five years or more performed worse on a series of cognitive tests than women who had used the drug for shorter periods (Paganini-Hill and Clark, 2001).

Raloxifene

Raloxifene is a nonsteroidal benzothiophen derivative that binds with high affinity to the nuclear ER (Baker et al., 1998; Brzozowski et al., 1997; Delmas et al., 1997; Yang et al., 1996). Like tamofen, raloxifene has a mixed pharmacological profile, acting as both ER agonist and antagonist in a tissue-specific manner (Brzozowski et al., 1997; Wijayaratne et al., 1999). In the breast and uterus, raloxifene acts as a classic antiestrogen to inhibit the growth of mammary or endometrial carcinoma (Purdie and Beardsworth, 1999), whereas in nonreproductive tissues it acts as a weak partial estrogen agonist to prevent bone loss and lower serum cholesterol levels (Baker et al., 1998; Delmas et al., 1997; Purdie and Beardsworth, 1999).

Studies conducted in neural preparations showed that raloxifene exerted mixed agonist/antagonist effects, mostly depending on the absence or presence of an ER full agonist. For example, in the rat hypothalamus, raloxifene alone increased dopamine content twofold, acting as a partial agonist; meanwhile, it was able to block the fivefold induction of dopamine levels by 17β-estradiol, acting as a full antagonist (Grandbois et al., 2000). Further, Genazzani and colleagues found that raloxifene exerted estrogen-like action on neuroendocrine opiatergic pathways when administered alone to ovariectomized rats, an effect that was reversed in fertile rats or in ovariectomized rats treated with 17β-estradiol, where it exerted an antiestrogen effect (Genazzani et al., 1999). Wu and colleagues, investigating the impact of raloxifene alone or in combination with 17β-estradiol on choline acetyltransferase activity, found that ovariectomized rats treated with either 17β-estradiol benzoate or raloxifene showed an increase in choline acetyltransferase activity (Wu et al., 1999). In studies using a rat pheochromocytoma cell line (PC12), raloxifene also showed estrogen agonist properties to increase process outgrowth when the PC12 cells were pretreated with nerve growth factor (Nilsen et al., 1998). In human females, raloxifene significantly increased hot flushes, suggesting that it acts as an ER antagonist on sites regulating vasomotor function (Cohen and Lu, 2000).

Studies in our laboratory sought to determine whether raloxifene exerted estrogen agonist or antagonist effects in hippocampal, cortical, and basal forebrain neurons. In low concentrations, raloxifene was modestly neuroprotective, comparable to other SERMs, and at a single concentration it increased the morphological complexity of hippocampal neurons but not of cortical and basal forebrain neurons. On the other hand, supraclinical concentrations of raloxifene were toxic to hippocampal and cortical neurons in culture. Further, in the presence of a postmenopausal level of 17β-estradiol, raloxifene functioned as a partial ER antagonist (O'Neill et al., 2004). These results indicate that raloxifene exerts partial to full estrogen agonist action in the absence of 17β-estradiol, whereas in the presence of 17β-estradiol, raloxifene exerts a mixed estrogen agonist/antagonist effect (O'Neill et al., 2004). The neuroprotective profile of raloxifene would predict that some beneficial effect would be achieved from clinically relevant doses of raloxifene but not from higher doses. It remains to be determined whether this magnitude of neuroprotection could lead to a decreased risk of developing AD, as has been shown with ET.

The Multiple Outcomes of Raloxifene Evaluation (MORE) trial, a randomized clinical trial of raloxifene in women with osteoporosis who also underwent cognitive testing, detected no differences between the raloxifene and placebo groups in the frequency of cognitive decline or in the occurrence of dementia. Both the raloxifene-treated group and the placebo group showed equal cognitive decline over the period of the study (Yaffe et al., 2001).

Clinical Implications

Together, the basic science and clinical research findings indicate that whereas currently available SERMs may be modest estrogen agonists in bone and effective antagonists in the breast and/or uterus, they are not effective estrogen agonists in the brain. Thus, the data indicate that neither soy-derived isoflavones nor tamoxifen nor raloxifene is effective at reversing the cognitive decline associated with menopause. These interventions would therefore not be expected to reduce the risk of AD in women.

The Development of NeuroSERMs for the Prevention of Neurodegenerative Disease

The goal of our NeuroSERM development efforts is to generate small-molecule therapeutics that easily penetrate the blood-brain barrier and that bind to mERs to activate estrogenic mechanisms that promote cognitive function and prevent age-associated neurodegenerative disease in both women and men (Brinton, 2002). Results from our laboratory and others have demonstrated that estrogen can activate a sequence of indirect genomic events that underlie estrogen promotion of memory function and protection against a series of neurodegenerative insults associated with AD. These basic scientific data not only provide insights into the mode of action of estrogen in the brain, they also serve as straightforward predictors for evaluating the therapeutic efficacy of other estrogen-like molecules in the brain. Our analyses of the impact of a series of ER ligands on neuronal function revealed that structurally variant estrogen alternatives possess both distinctive and overlapping pharmacological profiles in the brain. Based on these findings, we propose the design and development of effective alternative estrogen mimics that have the capability to activate the neurotrophic and neuroprotective mechanisms of estrogen in the brain while avoiding stimulation of reproductive organs. Our NeuroSERM design and development efforts have focused on computer-aided, structure-based drug design and discovery approaches. Following chemicoinformatic query of natural compound databases, 523 candidate molecules were identified, of which 60 showed in silico pharmacodynamic features required for activity and bioavailability necessary for a NeuroSERM. Based on our second design approach, we have designed 32 molecules that fulfill the molecular determinants for efficient binding with the ligand-binding pocket of either ERα or ERβ and have linked site-directed tail moieties to localize the molecule within the plasma membrane or to direct the molecule to mitochondria. Our efforts to develop a brain-selective estrogen, a NeuroSERM, not only should provide lead compounds but will also yield information on the unique requirements of the site of estrogen action necessary to promote and sustain neurological health while preventing the initial events that lead to neurodegenerative diseases such as AD.

Conclusions

Basic and clinical research findings combined have resulted in profoundly important insights into the efficacy of ET and HT in sustaining neurological health to prevent AD. The signaling cascades required for estrogen action in neurons provide a mechanistic understanding of why ET is efficacious for the prevention of AD but not for treating the disease. The calcium-dependent mechanism of estrogen action in neurons underlies the healthy-cell bias for estrogen-inducible proactive neuroprotection against degenerative insults and the promotion of morphogenesis in neurons. Our mechanistic understanding of estrogen action provides the foundation for developing effective therapeutics to promote neurological function and health throughout the menopausal years. To that end, we have begun a hybrid program of discovery and translational research to develop NeuroSERMs that promote the neurotrophic and neuroprotective benefits of estrogen in the brain while not inducing the adverse effects of estrogens. The goal of these efforts is to develop effective therapeutics with proactive defense and morphogenic benefits that could prevent age-related neurodegenerative diseases such as AD. The collaborative and interactive efforts of both basic and clinical scientists is central to the ultimate success of preventing the epidemic of AD.

ACKNOWLEDGMENTS

Work was supported by the National Institute on Aging, the National Institute of Mental Health, the Kenneth T. and Eileen L. Norris Foundation, the L. K. Whittier Foundation, the Stanley Family Trust, and the John Douglas French Foundation.

REFERENCES

Adams MM, Fink SE, Shah RA, et al. 2002. Estrogen and aging affect the subcellular distribution of estrogen receptor-alpha in the hippocampus of female rats. J Neurosci 22:3608–14.

Audesirk T, Cabell L, Kern M, et al. 2003. Beta-estradiol influences differentiation of hippocampal neurons in vitro through an estrogen receptor-mediated process. Neuroscience 121:927–34.

Baker VL, Draper M, Paul S, et al. 1998. Reproductive endocrine and endometrial effects of raloxifene hydrochloride, a selective estrogen receptor modulator, in women with regular menstrual cycles [see comments]. J Clin Endocrinol Metab 83:6–13.

Balabhadrapathruni S, Thomas TJ, Yurkow EJ, et al. 2000. Effects of genistein and structurally related phytoestrogens on cell cycle kinetics and apoptosis in MDA-MB-468 human breast cancer cells. Oncol Rep 7:3–12.

Bi R, Broutman G, Foy MR, et al. 2000. The tyrosine kinase and mitogen-activated protein kinase pathways mediate multiple effects of estrogen in hippocampus. Proc Natl Acad Sci USA 97:3602–7.

Bowers JL, Tyulmenkov VV, Jernigan SC, et al. 2000. Resveratrol acts as a mixed ago-
nist/antagonist for estrogen receptors alpha and beta. Endocrinology 141:3657–67.

Brinton RD. 1993. 17β-Estradiol induction of filopodial growth in cultured hippocampal neurons within minutes of exposure. Mol Cell Neurosci 4:36–46.

Brinton RD. 1999. A women's health issue: Alzheimer's disease and strategies for maintaining cognitive health. Int J Fertil Womens Med 44:174–85.

Brinton RD. 2001. Cellular and molecular mechanisms of estrogen regulation of memory function and neuroprotection against Alzheimer's disease: recent insights and
remaining challenges. Learn Mem 8:121–33.

Brinton RD. 2002. Selective estrogen receptor modulators (SERM) for the brain: recent
advances and remaining challenges for developing a NeuroSERM™. Drug Dev Res
56:380–92.

Brinton RD. 2004a. Estrogen therapy for prevention of Alzheimer's disease not for re-
habilitation following onset of disease: the healthy cell bias of estrogen action,
synaptic plasticity: from basic mechanisms to clinical applications. In *Synaptic Plasticity: Basic Mechanisms to Clinical Applications,* ed. M Baudry, X Bi, SS Schreiber,
131–37. New York: Taylor & Francis.

Brinton RD. 2004b. Impact of estrogen therapy on Alzheimer's disease: a fork in the
road? CNS Drugs 18:405–22.

Brinton RD, Nilsen J. 2001. Sex hormones and their brain receptors. In *International
Encyclopedia of the Social and Behavioral Sciences,* ed. NJ Smelser, PB Bates, 21:
13946–51. New York: Elsevier/Pergamon.

Brinton RD, Nilsen J. 2003. Effects of estrogen plus progestin on risk of dementia (com-
ment). JAMA 290:1707–9.

Brinton RD, Reichensperger JD, Brewer GJ. 2002. Estrogen regulation of age-related calcium dynamic in hippocampal neurons. Abstr Soc Neurosci 272.7.

Brinton RD, Tran J, Proffitt P, Montoya M. 1997. 17 beta-estradiol enhances the outgrowth and survival of neocortical neurons in culture. Neurochem Res 22:1339–51.

Brookmeyer R, Gray S, Kawas C. 1998. Projections of Alzheimer's disease in the United
States and the public health impact of delaying disease onset. Am J Public Health
88:1337–42.

Bruning PF. 1992. Droloxifene, a new anti-oestrogen in postmenopausal advanced
breast cancer: preliminary results of a double-blind dose-finding phase II trial. Eur J
Cancer 28A:1404–7.

Brzozowski AM, Pike AC, Dauter Z, et al. 1997. Molecular basis of agonism and antagonism in the oestrogen receptor. Nature 389:753–58.

Carlson MC, Zandi PP, Plassman BL, et al. 2001. Hormone replacement therapy and
reduced cognitive decline in older women: the Cache County Study. Neurology
57:2210–16.

Centers for Disease Control and Prevention. 2005. Available: www.cdc.gov/nchs/
fastats/hus/hus04trend.pdf#052.

Chen HY, Dykstra KD, Birzin ET, et al. 2004. Estrogen receptor ligands. Part 1. The discovery of flavanoids with subtype specificity. Bioorg Med Chem Lett 14:1417–22.

Chen HY, Kim S, Wu J, et al. 2004. Estrogen receptor ligands. Part 3. The SAR of dihydrobenzoxanthiin SERMs. Bioorg Med Chem Lett 14:2551–54.

Clodfelter GV, Porter NM, Landfield PW, et al. 2002. Sustained Ca(2+)-induced Ca(2+)-release underlies the post-glutamate lethal Ca(2+) plateau in older cultured hippocampal neurons. Eur J Pharmacol 447:189–200.

Coezy E, Borgna JL, Rochefort H. 1982. Tamoxifen and metabolites in MCF7 cells: correlation between binding to estrogen receptor and inhibition of cell growth. Cancer Res 42:317–23.

Cohen FJ, Lu Y. 2000. Characterization of hot flashes reported by healthy postmenopausal women receiving raloxifene or placebo during osteoporosis prevention trials. Maturitas 34:65–73.

Cole MP, Jones CT, Todd ID. 1971. A new anti-oestrogenic agent in late breast cancer: an early clinical appraisal of ICI46474. Br J Cancer 25:270–75.

Cordey M, Gundimeda U, Gopalakrishna R, et al. 2003. Estrogen activates protein kinase C in neurons: role in neuroprotection. J Neurochem 84:1340–48.

Couse JF, Lindzey J, Grandien K, et al. 1997. Tissue distribution and quantitative analysis of estrogen receptor-alpha (ERalpha) and estrogen receptor-beta (ERbeta) messenger ribonucleic acid in the wild-type and ERalpha-knockout mouse. Endocrinology 138:4613–21.

Datta SR, Dudek H, Tao X, et al. 1997. Akt phosphorylation of BAD couples survival signals to the cell-intrinsic death machinery. Cell 91:231–41.

Delmas PD, Bjarnason NH, Mitlak BH, et al. 1997. Effects of raloxifene on bone mineral density, serum cholesterol concentrations, and uterine endometrium in postmenopausal women. N Engl J Med 337:1641–47.

Dixon-Shanies D, Shaikh N. 1999. Growth inhibition of human breast cancer cells by herbs and phytoestrogens. Oncol Rep 6:1383–87.

Dubal DB, Zhu H, Yu J, et al. 2001. Estrogen receptor alpha, not beta, is a critical link in estradiol-mediated protection against brain injury. Proc Natl Acad Sci USA 98:1952–57.

Dykens JA, Simpkins JW, Wang J, et al. 2003. Polycyclic phenols, estrogens and neuroprotection: a proposed mitochondrial mechanism. Exp Gerontol 38:101–7.

Eppenberger U, Wosikowski K, Kung W. 1991. Pharmacologic and biologic properties of droloxifene, a new antiestrogen. Am J Clin Oncol 14:S5–14.

Espeland MA, Rapp SR, Shumaker SA, et al. 2004. Conjugated equine estrogens and global cognitive function in postmenopausal women: Women's Health Initiative Memory Study. JAMA 291:2959–68.

Fillit HM. 2000. The pharmacoeconomics of Alzheimer's disease. Am J Manag Care 6:S1139–44 [discussion S1145–38].

Fillit HM. 2002a. Economics, pharmacoeconomics and drug discovery for dementias. Drug Discov Today 7:785–87.

Fillit HM. 2002b. The role of hormone replacement therapy in the prevention of Alzheimer disease. Arch Intern Med 162:1934–42.

Fillit HM, O'Connell AW, Brown WM, et al. 2002. Barriers to drug discovery and development for Alzheimer disease. Alzheimer Dis Assoc Disord 16(Suppl 1):S1–8.

Foster TC. 2002. Regulation of synaptic plasticity in memory and memory decline with aging. Prog Brain Res 138:283–303.

Foster TC, Kumar A. 2002. Calcium dysregulation in the aging brain. Neuroscientist 8:297–301.

Foster TC, Sharrow KM, Kumar A, et al. 2003. Interaction of age and chronic estradiol replacement on memory and markers of brain aging. Neurobiol Aging 24:839–52.

Foy MR. 2001. 17beta-estradiol: effect on CA1 hippocampal synaptic plasticity. Neurobiol Learn Mem 76:239–52.

Foy MR, Xu J, Xie X, et al. 1999. 17β-estradiol enhances NMDA receptor-mediated EPSPs and long-term potentiation. J Neurophysiol 81:925–28.

Gao S, Hendrie HC, Hall KS, et al. 1998. The relationship between age, sex, and the incidence of dementia and Alzheimer disease: a meta-analysis. Arch Gen Psychiatry 55:809–15.

Genazzani AR, Bernardi F, Stomati M, et al. 1999. Raloxifene analog LY 117018: effects on central and peripheral beta-endorphin. Gynecol Endocrinol 13:249–58.

Gerber B, Krause A. 1999. New data concerning breast carcinoma: a report on the 34th meeting of the American Society of Clinical Oncology, Los Angeles, Calif., May 16–19, 1998. Gynakol Geburtshilfliche Rundsch 39:136–39.

Grandbois M, Morissette M, Callier S, et al. 2000. Ovarian steroids and raloxifene prevent MPTP-induced dopamine depletion in mice. Neuroreport 11:343–46.

Green PS, Gordon K, Simpkins JW. 1997. Phenolic A ring requirement for the neuroprotective effects of steroids. J Steroid Biochem Mol Biol 63:229–35.

Green PS, Yang SH, Nilsson KR, et al. 2001. The nonfeminizing enantiomer of 17beta-estradiol exerts protective effects in neuronal cultures and a rat model of cerebral ischemia. Endocrinology 142:400–406.

Grill HJ, Pollow K. 1991. Pharmacokinetics of droloxifene and its metabolites in breast cancer patients. Am J Clin Oncol 14:S21–29.

Guo J, Meng F, Fu X, et al. 2004. N-methyl-D-aspartate receptor and L-type voltage-gated Ca^{2+} channel activation mediate proline-rich tyrosine kinase 2 phosphorylation during cerebral ischemia in rats. Neurosci Lett 355:177–80.

Gust R, Keilitz R, Schmidt K, et al. 2002. (4R,5S)/(4S,5R)-4,5-Bis(4-hydroxyphenyl)-2-imidazolines: ligands for the estrogen receptor with a novel binding mode. J Med Chem 45:3356–65.

Hammond CB. 1994. Women's concerns with hormone replacement therapy: compliance issues. Fertil Steril 62(6 Suppl 2):157S–60S.

Henderson VW. 1997. The epidemiology of estrogen replacement therapy and Alzheimer's disease. Neurology 48:S27–35.

Henderson VW. 2000a. Hormone Therapy and the Brain: A Clinical Perspective on the Role of Estrogen. New York: Parthenon Publishing.

Henderson VW. 2000b. Oestrogens and dementia. Novartis Found Symp 230:254–65.

Henderson VW, Paganini-Hill A, Miller BL, et al. 2000. Estrogen for Alzheimer's disease in women: randomized, double-blind, placebo-controlled trial. Neurology 54:295–301.

Hogervorst E, Williams J, Budge M, et al. 2000. The nature of the effect of female gonadal hormone replacement therapy on cognitive function in post-menopausal women: a meta-analysis. Neurosci 101:485–512.

Hu XY, Qin S, Lu YP, et al. 2003. Decreased estrogen receptor-alpha expression in hippocampal neurons in relation to hyperphosphorylated tau in Alzheimer patients. Acta Neuropathol (Berl) 106:213–20.

Jordan VC. 2003a. Antiestrogens and selective estrogen receptor modulators as multifunctional medicines. 1. Receptor interactions. J Med Chem 46:883–908.

Jordan VC. 2003b. Antiestrogens and selective estrogen receptor modulators as multifunctional medicines. 2. Clinical considerations and new agents. J Med Chem 46: 1081–111.

Jordan VC, Collins MM, Rowsby L, et al. 1977. A monohydroxylated metabolite of tamoxifen with potent antioestrogenic activity. J Endocrinol 75:305–16.

Jordan VC, Koerner S. 1975. Tamoxifen (ICI 46,474) and the human carcinoma 8S oestrogen receptor. Eur J Cancer 11:205–6.

Kamada A, Sasaki A, Kitazawa N, et al. 2004. A new series of estrogen receptor modulators: effect of alkyl substituents on receptor-binding affinity. Chem Pharm Bull 52:79–88.

Katzenellenbogen BS, Sun J, Harrington WR, et al. 2001. Structure-function relationships in estrogen receptors and the characterization of novel selective estrogen receptor modulators with unique pharmacological profiles. Ann N Y Acad Sci 949:6–15.

Kawamura I, Mizota T, Kondo N, et al. 1991. Antitumor effects of droloxifene, a new antiestrogen drug, against 7,12-dimethylbenz(a)anthracene-induced mammary tumors in rats. Jpn J Pharmacol 57:215–24.

Kawas C, Resnick S, Morrison A, et al. 1997. A prospective study of estrogen replacement therapy and the risk of developing Alzheimer's disease: the Baltimore Longitudinal Study of Aging. Neurology 48:1517–21.

Kim MT, Brinton RD, Berger TW. 2002. Impact of estradiol on trisynaptic hippocampal circuit excitability using multisite electrode array. Abstr Soc Neurosci 272.6.

Kreijkamp-Kaspers S, Kok L, Grobbee DE, et al. 2004. Effect of soy protein containing isoflavones on cognitive function, bone mineral density, and plasma lipids in postmenopausal women: a randomized controlled trial. JAMA 292:65–74.

Kuroki Y, Fukushima K, Kanda Y, et al. 2000. Putative membrane-bound estrogen receptors possibly stimulate mitogen-activated protein kinase in the rat hippocampus. Eur J Pharmacol 400:205–9.

Kurzer MS, Xu X. 1997. Dietary phytoestrogens. Annu Rev Nutr 17:353–81.

LaFerla FM. 2002. Calcium dyshomeostasis and intracellular signalling in Alzheimer's disease. Nat Rev Neurosci 3:862–72.

LaFerla FM, Tinkle BT, Bieberich CJ, et al. 1995. The Alzheimer's A beta peptide induces neurodegeneration and apoptotic cell death in transgenic mice. Nat Genet 9:21–30.

Landfield PW. 1994. Increased hippocampal Ca^{2+} channel activity in brain aging and dementia: hormonal and pharmacologic modulation. Ann N Y Acad Sci 747:351–64.

Landfield PW, Thibault A, Mazzanti ML, et al. 1992. Mechanisms of neuronal death in brain aging and Alzheimer's disease: role of endocrine-mediated calcium dyshomeostasis. J Neurobiol 23:1247–60.

LeBlanc ES, Janowsky J, Chan BK, et al. 2001. Hormone replacement therapy and cognition: systematic review and meta-analysis. JAMA 285:1489–99.

Lee J, Brinton RD. 2003. Select protein kinase C isoforms regulate agonist-induced down-regulation of V1AR mRNA agonist-induced signal desensitization mechanism. Abstr Soc Neurosci 161.13.

Lee SJ, Campomanes CR, Sikat PT, et al. 2004. Estrogen induces phosphorylation of cyclic AMP response element binding (pCREB) in primary hippocampal cells in a time-dependent manner. Neuroscience 124:549–60.

Leissring MA, Paul BA, Parker I, et al. 1999. Alzheimer's presenilin-1 mutation potentiates inositol 1,4,5-triphosphate-mediated calcium signaling in *Xenopus* oocytes. J Neurochem 73:1061–68.

Lu YP, Zeng M, Hu XY, et al. 2003. Estrogen receptor alpha-immunoreactive astrocytes are increased in the hippocampus in Alzheimer's disease. Exp Neurol 183:482–88.

Lu YP, Zeng M, Swaab DF, et al. 2004. Colocalization and alteration of estrogen receptor-alpha and -beta in the hippocampus in Alzheimer's disease. Hum Pathol 35:275–80.

Makela S, Santti R, Salo L, et al. 1995. Phytoestrogens are partial estrogen agonists in the adult male mouse. Environ Health Perspect 103:123–27.

Manson JE, Hsia J, Johnson KC, et al. 2003. Estrogen plus progestin and the risk of coronary heart disease. N Engl J Med 349:523–34.

Masri R, Nilsen J, Irwin RW, et al. 2004. Estradiol-mediated mitochondrial regulation and neuroprotection. Abstr Soc Neurosci 659.4.

Mattson MP, Barger SW, Cheng B, et al. 1993. β-Amyloid precursor protein metabolites and loss of neuronal Ca^{2+} homeostasis in Alzheimer's disease. Trends Neurosci 16:409–14.

Mattson MP, LaFerla FM, Chan SL, et al. 2000. Calcium signaling in the ER: its role in neuronal plasticity and neurodegenerative disorders. Trends Neurosci 23:222–29.

McEwen B. 2002. Estrogen actions throughout the brain. Recent Prog Horm Res 57:357–84.

Migliaccio A, Di Domenico M, Castoria G, et al. 1996. Tyrosine kinase/p21ras/MAP-kinase pathway activation by estradiol-receptor complex in MCF-7 cells. EMBO J 15: 1292–1300.

Miller CP. 2002. SERMs: evolutionary chemistry, revolutionary biology. Curr Pharm Design 8:2089–111.

Miller CP, Collini MD, Tran BD, et al. 2001. Design, synthesis, and preclinical characterization of novel, highly selective indole estrogens. J Med Chem 44:1654–57.

Miller MM, Monjan AA, Buckholtz NS. 2001. Estrogen replacement therapy for the potential treatment or prevention of Alzheimer's disease. Ann N Y Acad Sci 949: 223–34.

Milner TA, McEwen BS, Hayashi S, et al. 2001. Ultrastructural evidence that hippocampal alpha estrogen receptors are located at extranuclear sites. J Comp Neurol 429:355–71.

Mitlak BH, Cohen FJ. 1997. In search of optimal long-term female hormone replacement: the potential of selective estrogen receptor modulators. Horm Res 48:155–63.

Mitra SW, Hoskin E, Yudkovitz J, et al. 2003. Immunolocalization of estrogen receptor beta in the mouse brain: comparison with estrogen receptor alpha. Endocrinology 144:2055–67.

Mulnard RA, Cotman CW, Kawas C, et al. 2000. Estrogen replacement therapy for treatment of mild to moderate Alzheimer disease: a randomized controlled trial. Alzheimer's Disease Cooperative Study [see comments]. JAMA 283:1007–15.

Nethrapalli IS, Singh M, Guan X, et al. 2001. Estradiol (E2) elicits SRC phosphorylation in the mouse neocortex: the initial event in E2 activation of the MAPK cascade? Endocrinology 142:5145–48.

Nilsen J, Brinton RD. 2002a. Impact of progestins on estradiol potentiation of the glutamate calcium response. Neuroreport 13:825–30.

Nilsen J, Brinton RD. 2002b. Impact of progestins on estrogen-induced neuroprotection: synergy by progesterone and 19-norprogesterone and antagonism by medroxyprogesterone acetate. Endocrinology 143:205–12.

Nilsen J, Brinton RD. 2003a. Mechanism of estrogen-mediated neuroprotection: regulation of mitochondial calcium and Bcl-2 expression. Proc Natl Acad Sci USA 100: 2842–47.

Nilsen J, Brinton RD. 2003b. Divergent impact of progesterone and medroxyprogesterone acetate (Provera) on nuclear mitogen-activated protein kinase signaling. Proc Natl Acad Sci USA 100:10506–11.

Nilsen J, Brinton RD. 2004. Mitochondria as therapeutic targets of estrogen action in the central nervous system. Curr Drug Targets CNS Neurol Disord 3:297–313.

Nilsen J, Chen S, Brinton RD. 2002. Dual action of estrogen on glutamate-induced calcium signaling: mechanisms requiring interaction between estrogen receptors and src/mitogen activated protein kinase pathway. Brain Res 930:216–34.

Nilsen J, Mor G, Naftolin F. 1998. Raloxifene induces neurite outgrowth in estrogen receptor positive PC12 cells. Menopause 5:211–16.

The North American Menopause Society. 2003. Menopause core curriculum study guide: basic overview, definitions, and statistics. Available on www.menopause.org (accessed March 9, 2003).

O'Neill K, Brinton RD. 2001. Impact of tamoxifen and its 4-hydroxy metabolite on neuronal correlates of memory and survival. Abstr Soc Neurosci 627.12.

O'Neill K, Brinton RD. 2002. The impact of tamoxifen and its 4-hydroxy metabolite on neuronal correlates of memory and survival. ENDO 2002 Abstracts, Annual Meeting of the Endocrine Society.

O'Neill K, Chen S, Brinton RD. 2004. Impact of the selective estrogen receptor modulator, raloxifene, on neuronal survival and outgrowth following toxic insults associated with aging and Alzheimer's disease. Exp Neurol 185:63–80.

Paganini-Hill A, Clark LJ. 2001. Preliminary assessment of cognitive function in breast cancer patients treated with tamoxifen. Breast Cancer Res Treat 64:165–76.

Pike CJ. 1999. Estrogen modulates neuronal Bcl-xL expression and beta-amyloid-induced apoptosis: relevance to Alzheimer's disease. J Neurochem 72:1552–63.

Porter NM, Landfield PW. 1998. Stress hormones and brain aging: adding injury to insult? Nat Neurosci 1:3–4.

Porter NM, Thibault O, Thibault V, et al. 1997. Calcium channel density and hippocampal cell death with age in long-term culture. J Neurosci 17:5629–39.

Purdie DW, Beardsworth SA. 1999. The selective oestrogen receptor modulation: evolution and clinical applications. Br J Clin Pharmacol 48:785–92.

Razandi M, Pedram A, Greene GL, et al. 1999. Cell membrane and nuclear estrogen receptors (ERs) originate from a single transcript: studies of ERalpha and ERbeta expressed in Chinese hamster ovary cells. Mol Endocrinol 13:307–19.

Renaud J, Bischoff SF, Buhl T, et al. 2003. Estrogen receptor modulators: identification and structure-activity relationships of potent ERalpha-selective tetrahydroisoquinoline ligands. J Med Chem 46:2945–57.

Rice M, Graves A, Larson E. 1995. Estrogen replacement therapy and cognition: role of phytoestrogens (abstr). Gerontologist 35(Suppl 1):169.

Sato M, Rippy MK, Bryant HU. 1996. Raloxifene, tamoxifen, nafoxidine, or estrogen effects on reproductive and nonreproductive tissues in ovariectomized rats. FASEB J 10:905–12.

Savaskan E, Olivieri G, Meier F, et al. 2001. Hippocampal estrogen beta-receptor immunoreactivity is increased in Alzheimer's disease. Brain Res 908:113–19.

Shang Y, Brown M. 2002. Molecular determinants for the tissue specificity of SERMs. Science 295:2465–68.

Shi J, Bui JD, Yang SH, et al. 2001. Estrogens decrease reperfusion-associated cortical ischemic damage: an MRI analysis in a transient focal ischemia model. Stroke 32:987–92.

Shughrue PJ, Merchenthaler I. 2000. Evidence for novel estrogen binding sites in the rat hippocampus. Neuroscience 99:605–12.

Shughrue PJ, Scrimo PJ, Merchenthaler I. 2000. Estrogen binding and estrogen receptor characterization (ERalpha and ERbeta) in the cholinergic neurons of the rat basal forebrain. Neuroscience 96:41–49.

Shumaker SA, Legault C, Kuller L, et al. 2004. Conjugated equine estrogens and incidence of probable dementia and mild cognitive impairment in postmenopausal women: Women's Health Initiative Memory Study. JAMA 291:2947–58.

Shumaker SA, Legault C, Rapp SR, et al. 2003. Estrogen plus progestin and the incidence of dementia and mild cognitive impairment in postmenopausal women: the Women's Health Initiative Memory Study: a randomized controlled trial. JAMA 289:2651–62.

Simoncini T, Hafezi-Moghadam A, Brazil DP, et al. 2000. Interaction of oestrogen receptor with the regulatory subunit of phosphatidylinositol-3-OH kinase. Nature 407:538–41.

Singer CA, Figueroa-Masot XA, Batchelor RH, et al. 1999. The mitogen-activated protein kinase pathway mediates estrogen neuroprotection after glutamate toxicity in primary cortical neurons. J Neurosci 19:2455–63.

Singer CA, Rogers KL, Dorsa DM. 1998. Modulation of Bcl-2 expression: a potential component of estrogen protection in NT2 neurons. Neuroreport 9:2565–68.

Singh AK. 2001. Development of QSAR models to predict estrogenic, carcinogenic, and cancer protective effects of phytoestrogens. Cancer Invest 19:201–16.

Singh M. 2001. Ovarian hormones elicit phosphorylation of Akt and extracellular-signal regulated kinase in explants of the cerebral cortex. Endocr J 14:407–15.

Singh M, Meyer EM, Millard WJ, et al. 1994. Ovarian steroid deprivation results in a reversible learning impairment and compromised cholinergic function in female Sprague-Dawley rats. Brain Res 644:305–12.

Singh M, Setalo G Jr, Guan X, et al. 1999. Estrogen-induced activation of mitogen-activated protein kinase in cerebral cortical explants: convergence of estrogen and neurotrophin signaling pathways. J Neurosci 19:1179–88.

Singh M, Setalo G Jr, Guan X, et al. 2000. Estrogen-induced activation of the mitogen-activated protein kinase cascade in the cerebral cortex of estrogen receptor-alpha knock-out mice. J Neurosci 20:1694–1700.

Stahl S, Chun TY, Gray WG. 1998. Phytoestrogens act as estrogen agonists in an estrogen-responsive pituitary cell line. Toxicol Appl Pharmacol 152:41–48.

Tang MX, Jacobs D, Stern Y, et al. 1996. Effect of oestrogen during menopause on risk and age at onset of Alzheimer's disease. Lancet 348:429–32.

Thibault A, Hadley R, Landfield PW. 2001. Elevated postsynaptic Ca[2+]i and L-type calcium channel activity in aged hippocampal neurons: relationship to impaired synaptic plasticity. J Neurosci 21:9744–56.

Thibault A, Landfield PW. 1996. Increase in single L-type calcium channels in hippocampal neurons during aging. Science 272:1017–20.

Thibault O, Porter NM, Chen KC, et al. 1998. Calcium dysregulation in neuronal aging and Alzheimer's disease: history and new directions. Cell Calcium 24:417–33.

Thomas SM, Brugge JS. 1997. Cellular functions regulated by Src family kinases. Annu Rev Cell Dev Biol 13:513–609.

Tice JA, Ettinger B, Ensrud K, et al. 2003. Phytoestrogen supplements for the treatment of hot flashes: the Isoflavone Clover Extract (ICE) Study: a randomized controlled trial. JAMA 290:207–14.

Toran-Allerand CD. 2004. Minireview: A plethora of estrogen receptors in the brain: where will it end? Endocrinology 145:1069–74.

Wang C, Kurzer MS. 1997. Phytoestrogen concentration determines effects on DNA synthesis in human breast cancer cells. Nutr Cancer 28:236–47.

Watanabe N, Ikeno A, Minato H, et al. 2003. Discovery and preclinical characterization of (+)-3-[4-(1-piperidinoethoxy)phenyl]spiro[indene-1,1'-indane]-5,5'-diol hydrochloride: a promising nonsteroidal estrogen receptor agonist for hot flush. J Med Chem 46:3961–64.

Waters KM, Rickard DJ, Riggs BL, et al. 2001. Estrogen regulation of human osteoblast function is determined by the stage of differentiation and the estrogen receptor isoform. J Cell Biochem 83:448–62.

Watson CS, Campbell CH, Gametchu B. 2002. The dynamic and elusive membrane estrogen receptor-alpha. Steroids 67:429–37.

Watson CS, Pappas TC, Gametchu B. 1995. The other estrogen receptor in the plasma membrane: implications for the actions of environmental estrogens. Environ Health Perspect 103(Suppl 7):41–50.

Watters JJ, Campbell JS, Cunningham MJ, et al. 1997. Rapid membrane effects of steroids in neuroblastoma cells: effects of estrogen on mitogen activated protein kinase signalling cascade and c-fos immediate early gene transcription. Endocrinology 138:4030–33.

Whitehouse PJ. 1997. Alzheimer's disease: an international public health problem. Clinical goals, strategies, and outcomes. In *Pharmacological Treatment of Alzheimer's Disease*, ed. JD Brioni, MW Decker, 331–43. New York: Wiley Liss.

Wijayaratne AL, Nagel SC, Paige LA, et al. 1999. Comparative analyses of mechanistic differences among antiestrogens. Endocrinology 140:5828–40.

Wise PM, Dubal DB, Wilson ME, et al. 2001. Estradiol is a protective factor in the adult and aging brain: understanding of mechanisms derived from in vivo and in vitro studies. Brain Res Rev 37:313–19.

Woolley CS. 1999. Electrophysiological and cellular effects of estrogen on neuronal function. Crit Rev Neurobiol 13:1–20.

Woolley CS, McEwen BS. 1994. Estradiol regulates hippocampal dendritic spine density via an N-methyl-D-aspartate receptor-dependent mechanism. J Neurosci 14:7680–87.

Wu T, Wang J, Brinton RD. 2003. 17β-Estradiol activation of L-type Ca^{2+} channels is required for transcriptional cascade leading to neuroprotection. Abstr Soc Neurosci 504.12.

Wu TW, Wang JM, Chen S, et al. 2005. 17β-Estradiol induced Ca^{2+} influx via L-type calcium channels activates the Src/Erk/CREB signal pathway and bcl-2 expression in rat hippocampal neurons: a potential initiation mechanism for estrogen-induced neuroprotection. Neuroscience 135:59–72.

Wu X, Glinn MA, Ostrowski NL, et al. 1999. Raloxifene and estradiol benzoate both fully restore hippocampal choline acetyltransferase activity in ovariectomized rats. Brain Res 847:98–104.

Wymann MP, Pirola L. 1998. Structure and function of phosphoinositide 3-kinases. Biochim Biophys Acta 1436:127–50.

Yaffe K, Krueger K, Sarkar S, et al. 2001. Cognitive function in postmenopausal women treated with raloxifene. N Engl J Med 344:1207–13.

Yaffe K, Sawaya G, Lieberburg I, et al. 1998. Estrogen therapy in postmenopausal women: effects on cognitive function and dementia. JAMA 279:688–95.

Yang C, Edsall R Jr, Harris HA, et al. 2004. ERbeta ligands. Part 2. Synthesis and structure-activity relationships of a series of 4-hydroxy-byphenyl-carbaldehyde oxime derivatives. Bioorg Med Chem 12:2553–70.

Yang NN, Bryant HU, Hardikar S, et al. 1996. Estrogen and raloxifene stimulate transforming growth factor–beta 3 gene expression in rat bone: a potential mechanism for estrogen- or raloxifene-mediated bone maintenance. Endocrinology 137:2075–84.

Yang SH, Liu R, Perez EJ, et al. 2004. Mitochondrial localization of estrogen receptor beta. Proc Natl Acad Sci USA 101:4130–35.

Zandi PP, Anthony JC, Hayden KM, et al. 2002. Reduced incidence of AD with NSAID but not H$_2$ receptor antagonists: the Cache County Study. Neurology 59:880–86.

Zandi PP, Carlson MC, Plassman BL, et al. 2002. Hormone replacement therapy and incidence of Alzheimer disease in older women: the Cache County Study. JAMA 288: 2123–29.

Zava DT, Duwe G. 1997. Estrogenic and antiproliferative properties of genistein and other flavonoids in human breast cancer cells in vitro. Nutr Cancer 27:31–40.

Zhao L, Brinton RD. 2002. Neuroprotective and neurotrophic efficacy of phytoestrogens in cultured hippocampal neurons. Exp Neurol 227:509–19.

Zhao L, Chen S, Ming Wang J, et al. 2005. 17Beta-estradiol induces Ca^{2+} influx, dendritic and nuclear Ca^{2+} rise and subsequent cyclic AMP response element-binding protein activation in hippocampal neurons: a potential initiation mechanism for estrogen neurotrophism. Neuroscience 132:299–311.

Zhao L, Wu T-W, Brinton RD. 2004. Estrogen receptor subtypes alpha and beta contribute to neuroprotection and increased Bcl-2 expression in primary hippocampal neurons. Brain Res 101:22–34.

Znamensky V, Akama KT, McEwen BS, et al. 2003. Estrogen levels regulate the subcellular distribution of phosphorylated Akt in hippocampal CA1 dendrites. J Neurosci 23:2340–47.

CHAPTER 6

Basic and Clinical Data on the Effects of SERMs on Cognition

KRISTINE YAFFE, M.D., PAULINE M. MAKI, Ph.D.,
AND PETER J. SCHMIDT, M.D.

At least 10 percent of persons over 65 years old and 50 percent of those over 85 have some form of cognitive impairment, ranging from mild deficits to dementia (Evans, 1990). Alzheimer disease (AD), the most common cause of dementia, is currently estimated to affect 4 million people in the United States and to cost $70 billion annually, but it is projected to affect vastly more—14 million—by the year 2040 (Brookmeyer et al., 1998). AD affects women disproportionately, with women having a slightly increased risk of AD, even after adjusting for age (Launer et al., 1999). Despite the severity and prevalence of dementia and mild cognitive impairment, there are few effective treatments or prevention strategies.

Estrogen Therapy and the Risk of Developing AD and Other Dementias

Estrogen therapy (ET) has been one of the most compelling potential strategies for the prevention of dementia, primarily AD. There is strong biological evidence of estrogen's beneficial effects on the brain, including neurotrophic effects, reductions in β-amyloid accumulation, enhanced neurotransmitter release and action, and protection against oxidative damage (McEwen, 1999; Xu et al., 1998).

Data from the recently terminated Women's Health Initiative Memory Study (WHIMS), however, failed to find a benefit of combined estrogen plus progestin therapy (0.625 mg/day of conjugated estrogen and 2.5 mg/day of medroxyprogesterone acetate) on the risk of developing dementia. Indeed, in this ancillary study of 4,532 women 65 years old or older, hormone treatment (HT) for four years resulted in an approximately twofold higher incidence of dementia (hazard ratio = 2.05, 95% confidence interval [CI]: 1.21–3.48) (Shumaker et al., 2003). Although the number of women with dementia was small, the data suggest that HT increased the risk for all types of dementia. The results of the estrogen-alone arm of WHIMS also failed to support a protective effect of estrogen on the development of all-cause dementia (Shumaker et al., 2004). These results, along with those from the main WHI trial, highlight that the harm of HT outweighs the benefits and that HT should be reserved for the treatment of menopausal symptoms and should not be used for the prevention of disease, including dementia.

Selective Estrogen Receptor Modulators

Estrogen's myriad effects in the central nervous system (CNS), and observational data suggesting a beneficial role of estrogen on cognition and in the prevention of dementia, have led to increasing interest in new estrogen-like agents. Selective estrogen receptor modulators (SERMs) are the founding members of a class of pharmacological agents that bind to nuclear hormone receptors and display a differential pattern of activities relative to the parent ligand. SERMs are ER ligands that act as either partial agonists or antagonists, and the selective quality of these compounds has traditionally referred to their tissue-specific actions relative to those of estradiol (Jordan, 2003). For example, SERMs may act like estradiol in one tissue (e.g., bone) but not in another (e.g., endometrium). They also have the potential to display differential affinities and selectivity for ER subtypes α and β (Katzenellenbogen and Katzenellenbogen, 2000). The mechanisms underlying the tissue-specific actions of SERMs relative to estradiol and the exact mechanism whereby the actions of individual SERMs vary within the same tissue have not been investigated fully. Elucidation of the mechanism of action of SERMs should help answer a central question about the biological effects of estrogen, namely, how can the actions of estrogen be turned on or off in a given tissue to select a desired physiological outcome? Not surprisingly, much of our understanding of the mechanism of actions of SERMs has been informed by the known complexities of ER-ligand interactions and transcriptional effects.

The ER is a modular protein (Lonard and Smith, 2002; Tsai and O'Malley, 1994) containing specific regions in its structure that are responsible for several activities, including ligand and DNA binding, as well as at least two trans-activating functions (TAF-1 and TAF-2). The traditional model of estrogen's genomic action involves the entry of estrogen into the cell, where it binds the ligand-binding domain of the ER; the receptor undergoes phosphorylation, release from heat-shock proteins, and dimer formation; and the DNA-binding domain of ER interacts with the estrogen response element (ERE) within the promoter of the responsive gene. Interactions between the ligand-ER-DNA complex and coregulator proteins (coactivators, corepressors) modulate the amount of transcriptional activity. For example, coactivators facilitate transcription by remodeling/unfolding chromatin, acetylating histones, and regulating transcription reinitiation activities (Jones and Kadonaga, 2000; Lonard and Smith, 2002; McKenna and O'Malley, 2002; Smith and O'Malley, 2004), whereas corepressors may inhibit ER-ligand binding, as well as interfere with transcription at the ERE (e.g., by deacetylating histones) (Nagy et al., 1997; Smith and O'Malley, 2004).

Several additional factors influence ER-mediated transcriptional activity and may contribute to tissue specificity. The first is the relative proportions of the ER subtypes. ERα and ERβ (and their variants) may combine to form heterodimers and differentially regulate transcription (Pettersson et al., 2000). ERβ inhibits ERα in some tissues, and therefore the tissue-specific localization of ER isoforms could modulate the observed effect of a ligand across different tissues. Second, the amount of coactivator and corepressor binding is regulated in part by the specific types and amounts of these proteins available within the cell and by their rates of synthesis and degradation. Additionally, the structural conformation of the ligand-binding domain changes in response to the size and shape of the ligand to promote (agonists) or inhibit (antagonists) coactivator binding. Finally, the presence of cointegrator proteins allows ERs to activate transcription at AP1 (SP1) sites in the absence of an ERE on the responsive gene (Webb et al., 1995). The mechanisms involved in ER-ligand-ERE interactions are part of an extremely complex physiological system, and there is considerable potential for variability in both the signaling process and the observed tissue effects. For example, the phosphorylation or substitution of a single amino acid within ERα will influence the structure of the ER-ligand complex sufficiently to alter the relative agonist or antagonist action expressed by the same ligand within a tissue (Jensen and Jordan, 2003). Finally, the effects of estradiol within a given tissue, including the CNS, are context-specific and may differ depending on such variables as age, gender, genetics, level of stress, presence of pathology, and developmental stage (Rubinow et al., 2002).

Both the therapeutic and the conceptual importance of SERMs are defined by the tissue-dependent nature of their estrogen-like effects. The effect of a SERM on ER-regulated transcription differs according to whether the SERM behaves as an agonist, and therefore mimics estrogen's binding and subsequent transcriptional activity, or as an antagonist. Moreover, these actions vary from one type of SERM to another. As agonists, SERMs bind to the ER and initiate the sequence of events (e.g., coactivator recruitment) leading to transcription, similar to the sequence described for estrogen. In contrast, in tissues in which antagonist actions predominate, the SERM binds to the ligand-binding domain, and the ER-SERM configuration inhibits coactivator binding and may promote corepressor binding (Pike et al., 1999; Smith and O'Malley, 2004). SERMs have differential actions in relation to ERα and ERβ both in their ability to alter the binding of cofactors and in their binding affinities (Kuiper et al., 1997). Although raloxifene can act as a partial agonist with ERα, in the presence of estradiol it has a 15-fold greater inhibition at ERα than at ERβ. Tamoxifen, on the other hand, inhibits ERα and ERβ equally (Barkhem et al., 1998). Indeed, most of the currently available SERMs display little agonist activity with ERβ (Barkhem et al., 1998), although some ERβ-selective agonists are being developed (Harris et al., 2003; Yang et al., 2004). Individual tissues may have a specific profile of coregulators that influence whether the SERM acts as an agonist or as an antagonist. For example, the presence of higher levels of steroid receptor coactivator 1 in uterine cancer cells compared with breast cancer cells was associated with tamoxifen's agonist action in the former but not the latter tissue (Shang and Brown, 2002). Within normal tissues, however, the relevance of differing coregulator concentrations to the tissue-specific effects of SERMs remains to be demonstrated (McDonnell and Norris, 2002; Smith and O'Malley, 2004).

Like estrogen, SERMs have been reported to bind membrane-bound ER, induce coactivator expression, influence the process of ubiquitinization and proteasome activity, and interact (like estrogen) with cointegrators at both the AP1 and SP1 sites (i.e., independent of EREs) (Smith and O'Malley, 2004).

Raloxifene and estradiol bind to ERα or ERβ, and the resulting complexes have distinct actions at the AP1-binding site (Paech et al., 1997), with estradiol inhibiting and raloxifene stimulating AP1 transcriptional activities when bound to ERβ and estradiol stimulating transcription at AP1 when bound to ERα. Obviously, many factors (Jensen and Jordan, 2003) modify SERM-ER actions within the cell and potentially explain the observed tissue specificity of these compounds. Nevertheless, the ability to dissect out the effects of SERMs within selected tissues should allow new compounds to be developed as alternatives to estrogen.

Thus, SERMs provide the opportunity to target estrogen-like effects within certain tissues, improve the long-term safety profile of HT, and, possibly, modulate the magnitude of an estrogenic effect within specific tissues (e.g., by reducing competitive inhibition across receptor subtypes). Alternatively, SERMs could be coadministered with estrogen to counteract unwanted side effects (Labrie et al., 2003).

Genetics of the Estrogen Receptor and Effects on Cognition

Several genes associated with familial and sporadic AD have been identified, but it is estimated that roughly half of the genetic factors remain unidentified (Brandi et al., 1999). Recent genetic research has focused on identifying common population polymorphism loci, such as apolipoprotein E (APOE) and α_1-antichymotrypsin, that are associated with an increased susceptibility to AD. We address the evidence that sex hormone receptor gene variants or polymorphisms may be associated with a risk of AD and cognitive decline in older men and women.

Ovariectomized ERα knockout mice have impaired performance on a hippocampal-dependent cognitive task that is reversed with estradiol administration (Fugger et al., 2000). The abundant localization of ERβ in human hippocampus supports a role for this receptor in cognition as well (Osterlund et al., 2000; Savaskan et al., 2001). The density of ERβ has been reported to be increased in the brains of persons with AD compared to elderly controls (Savaskan et al., 2001).

The ERα gene polymorphism is a possible candidate for AD susceptibility in sporadic AD. Several studies have shown that ET improves cognitive function or prevents AD in elderly women (Kawas et al., 1997; Resnick et al., 1997; Sherwin, 1988; Tang et al., 1996) and that women have a slightly higher age-adjusted risk of developing AD than men, possibly mediated by the APOE genotype (Farrer et al., 1997). The gene for ERα has several single nucleotide polymorphisms (SNPs), the PvuII, XbaI, and B variants, that may be associated with receptor expression and function (Albagha et al., 2001; Maruyama et al., 2000). Although the finding is controversial, differences in ERβ polymorphism frequencies have been demonstrated in several diseases, including breast cancer, osteoporosis, and endometriosis (Anderson et al., 1997; Deng et al., 1999; Georgiou et al., 1999). Several case-control studies (Brandi et al., 1999; Isoe-Wada et al., 1999; Mattila et al., 2000), but not all (Maruyama et al., 2000), found an increased frequency of the PvuII and XbaI polymorphisms (polymorphic sites that are in linkage disequilibrium) in patients with AD compared to controls. Furthermore, a case-control study reported a synergistic effect of ERβ CA repeat polymorphism and ERα PvuII and XbaI polymorphisms on the risk of developing AD in older white individuals (Lambert et al., 2001).

The association among ERα polymorphisms, cognitive test performance, and risk of cognitive impairment and dementia in community-dwelling older women of European ancestry was investigated as part of a prospective study (Yaffe et al., 2002). The subjects for the study were 2,625 women without dementia who underwent cognitive testing at baseline and at six to eight years of follow-up. The frequency of PvuII genotypes among the women was 21% (n = 549) with PP, 46% (n = 1,217) with Pp, and 33% (n = 859) with pp. The frequency of the XbaI genotype was 12% (n = 315) with XX, 47% (n = 1,232) with Xx, and 31% (n = 1,078) with xx. The decline in cognitive performance from baseline to testing six to eight years later was greater in women with at least one p allele compared with women without a p allele (P for trend = 0.01) and in women with at least one x allele compared with women without an x allele (P for trend = 0.02) when the analyses were adjusted for age, education, and baseline score.

ERα allele frequencies differed among women who developed cognitive impairment compared to those who did not, with more women who developed cognitive impairment having a p allele (62% versus 56%, P = 0.03; age- and education-adjusted odds ratio [OR] = 1.35, 95% CI: 1.07–1.72). Similarly, more women who developed cognitive impairment had an x allele (70% versus 64%, P = 0.03; OR = 1.32, 95% CI: 1.03–1.68). Among the 62 women who said they had received a diagnosis of dementia or AD from their physician, the gene frequency for p was 65 percent (P = 0.03 compared to those without a diagnosis of dementia), and for x it was 74 percent (P = 0.02). ERα genotype frequencies also differed among women who did and did not develop cognitive impairment. Using the PP genotype as a reference, women who had a pp or Pp genotype had an increased likelihood of developing cognitive impairment (OR = 1.65, 95% CI: 1.03–2.63 for pp, and OR = 1.32, 95% CI: 0.84–2.09 for Pp). Similarly, the adjusted odds of developing impairment were higher in women with the xx genotype but not in women with the Xx genotype compared with women with the XX genotype (age- and education-adjusted OR = 1.73, 95% CI: 0.99–3.02 for xx; adjusted OR = 1.17, 95% CI: 0.66–2.06 for Xx). Compared to women with PP or XX, the age- and education-adjusted odds of receiving a physician's diagnosis of dementia or AD were increased by almost threefold among women with pp (adjusted OR = 2.68, 95% CI: 1.14–6.31) or xx (adjusted OR = 3.06, 95% CI:1.06–8.83).

Although the polymorphisms may affect ERα gene enhancer activity (Maruyama et al., 2000) or gene regulation (Albagha et al., 2001), in vitro evidence indicates that the ERα PvuII polymorphism produces a functional myb transcription factor binding site, suggesting that it produces a novel promoter or intronic enhancer of ERα expression (Herrington et al., 2002). How the ERα polymorphisms may influence cognitive function is not known. It may be, for example, that ER polymorphisms are associated with different estradiol serum concentrations, which in turn may predict cognitive decline (Yaffe, Lui, et al., 2000). Studies have described an interaction between the ERα polymorphisms and APOE ε4 allele on the risk of developing AD (Mattila et al., 2000). The observed interaction between APOE ε4 and oral ET on the risk of developing cognitive impairment also supports the hypothesis that estrogen, and possibly ERα polymorphisms, and APOE may be mechanistically linked in their effect on cognitive decline (Yaffe, Haan, et al., 2000). Several lines of evidence from in vitro and animal studies, including estradiol-induced synaptic sprouting and expression of APOE mRNA in rodents, support an estrogen-APOE interaction (Srivastava et al., 1997; Stone et al., 1998). It is also possible that the increased risk of cognitive impairment observed with the ERα polymorphisms is due to linkage disequilibrium with nearby genes, which may in turn cause an increased risk of developing AD or other dementias.

If sex hormones play a role in the prevention of AD and other cognitive decline, it is likely that genetic variations in sex hormone receptors and metabolic genes are linked to risk of AD and cognitive decline. Preliminary data support an association between several ERα polymorphisms and the risk of AD and cognitive decline in older women. Further research should determine the mechanism for this association.

Estrogen Receptor Activity, SERMs, and the CNS

ERs are widely distributed within the brain, and both ERα and ERβ (as well as some of their variants) have been identified in brain regions involved in the regulation of mood, cognition, and behavior. Estrogen, acting through ERα and ERβ, regulates many aspects of both neuronal and glial cell function considered relevant to the regulation of mood, cognition, and behavior in humans. Disorders of both mood and cognition are associated with abnormalities of neurotransmitter and neuropeptide systems, including those regulated by serotonin, -γ-aminobutyric acid (GABA), N-methyl-D-aspartate (NMDA), dopamine, and acetylcholine. Estrogen's effects in these systems are considerable and involve the production of synthetic and degradative enzymes, the regulation of receptor density and binding, and transporter activity (McEwen, 2002). Alternatively, studies suggest a role for cyclic AMP response element-binding protein (CREB) and brain-derived neurotrophic factor (BDNF) in the pathophysiology and treatment of these disorders (Duman et al., 1997; Murer et al., 2001; Tully et al., 2003). Estrogen has been reported to increase BDNF in the forebrain and hippocampus (Singh et al., 1995; Sohrabji, Miranda, et al., 1994) and to increase CREB and trkA in rat (Panickar et al., 1997; Sohrabji, Greene, et al., 1994; Zhou et al., 1996), consistent with putative antidepressant and memory-enhancing effects. Indeed, estrogen has been observed to modulate neuronal plasticity through dendritic spine and synapse formation, as well as glial activity, in several brain regions, including the hippocampus and prefrontal cortex. Finally, estrogen demonstrates a neuroprotective action in several models of neurotoxicity.

Despite the ability of many SERMs to cross the blood-brain barrier, only a few studies have examined the effects of SERMs on brain function. Observations to date suggest that, with the exception of the hypothalamus, short-term administration of SERMs has similar effects on the CNS to those observed after estrogen administration. Both raloxifene and estrogen have been observed to display nerve growth factor–like neurotrophic actions in cultured PC12 cells, with both compounds promoting neurite growth (Nilsen et al., 1998). Similarly, raloxifene promotes neurite outgrowth in cultured mouse hippocampal cells (but not cortical or basal forebrain cells) in a manner similar to estrogen, with outgrowth blocked by an NMDA receptor antagonist (O'Neill et al., 2004). In contrast to estrogen, high doses of raloxifene were neurotoxic in this study (O'Neill et al., 2004). Estrogen-induced neurite outgrowth and dendritic spine formation may be mediated by alterations in BDNF (Murphy et al., 1998) or NMDA (McEwen, 2002) receptor actions. Raloxifene also increases BDNF mRNA in the CA3 region of the hippocampus and frontal cortex (Wu et al., 1999), and both raloxifene and tamoxifen decrease AMPA-specific binding in the frontal cortex and striatum (Cyr, Morissette, et al., 2001) of ovariectomized rats in a manner qualitatively similar to that observed after ET. Moreover, the effects of raloxifene and tamoxifen in preventing the ovariectomy-induced decrease in NMDA receptor binding and NR subunit mRNA expression within the hippocampus of rats are similar to those observed after estradiol treatment (Cyr, Thibault, et al., 2001).

In addition to their effects on spine formation and possibly neuroplasticity, SERMs modulate many of the neurotransmitter systems in a manner similar to estrogen. In ovariectomized rats, both raloxifene and estradiol reversed ovariectomy-induced decreases in choline acetyltransferase (ChAT) activity in the hippocampus (Wu et al., 1999). The ability of ET to increase hippocampal ChAT activity in ovariectomized rats has a functional correlate, and is associated with improved performance on a passive avoidance memory task (Singh et al., 1994). However, raloxifene did not have similar beneficial effects to those of estradiol on a spatial working memory task administered to aged, ovariectomized rhesus monkeys (Lacreuse et al., 2002). Similarly, estrogen exerts manifold actions on the serotonergic system, and both raloxifene and estradiol increase 5-HT2A receptor density and expression in cingulate and frontal cortices, striatum, and nucleus accumbens of ovariectomized rats (Cyr et al., 2000). Additionally, Bethea et al. (2002) documented that estradiol, raloxifene, and arzoxifene have similar effects on measures of serotonergic system function, including increased tryptophan hydroxylase mRNA, decreased SERT mRNA, and no effect on 5-HT1A message in the midbrain of ovariectomized rhesus macaques. In rodents, however, raloxifene did not alter SERT mRNA in the midbrain, amygdala, or hypothalamus (Zhou et al., 2002). Finally, a potential neuroprotective role for SERMs has been suggested by the following reports: raloxifene, estradiol, and progesterone prevent MPTP-induced dopamine depletion in mouse striatum (Callier et al., 2001; Grandbois et al., 2000); long-term (60-day) exposure to either raloxifene or estrogen significantly lowered the numbers of astrocytes and microglia in the hippocampus of aging ovariectomized female mice compared with placebo-treated animals (Lei et al., 2003); and raloxifene demonstrated neuroprotective effects in several models of neurotoxicity, although the magnitude of neuroprotection varied for each toxin in a brain region–specific manner and was comparable to that of estradiol only in the context of free radical toxicity induced by hydrogen peroxide (O'Neill et al., 2004). In contrast to the majority of these reports, in rats, raloxifene antagonizes estrogen induction of both progesterone receptor mRNA in the preoptic area (Shughrue et al., 1997) and lordotis behavior (Meisel et al., 1987). Thus, because of raloxifene's action in the hypothalamus, it is more commonly characterized as an estrogen receptor antagonist.

The similarity between the neuromodulatory effects of many of the existing SERMs and estrogen's effects predicts that SERMs would have effects on cognition and mood similar to those of estrogen. However, the differential actions of SERMs on ERβ or the brain region–specific effects of SERMs, for example, may be sufficient to significantly alter the response compared to that for estrogen.

SERMs and Cognition in Women

The two FDA-approved SERMS are tamoxifen and raloxifene. Both have estrogen agonist properties in bone and lipids and estrogen antagonist effects in the breast, while raloxifene, unlike tamoxifen, has estrogen antagonist effects in the uterus (Draper et al., 1996). The identification of ERs in multiple brain regions, along with the recognition that SERMs have differential tissue-dependent effects on ER function, has prompted interest in the effects of raloxifene and other SERMs on cognition.

To date, there are no published trials of the effects of tamoxifen on objective measures of cognitive function or dementia outcomes. Two trials, however, have examined subjective cognitive complaints. One trial, conducted in 293 premenopausal breast cancer patients who had undergone adjuvant chemotherapy, found no differences in subjective cognitive complaints among groups of women randomly assigned to goserelin, goserelin plus tamoxifen, tamoxifen alone, or no endocrine therapy for two years (Nystedt et al., 2003). By contrast, a study of 2,653 postmenopausal breast cancer patients found that compared with nonusers, a greater proportion of women who had used tamoxifen reported seeing their physicians for memory problems (Paganini-Hill and Clark, 2001).

Three observational studies examined the impact of tamoxifen on objective cognitive test performance in women with a history of breast cancer. One compared cognitive performance on three tests among women with a history of breast cancer, some of whom had previously taken tamoxifen (Schagen et al., 1999). There were no statistically significant differences on the cognitive test scores between those previously exposed to tamoxifen and those without previous exposure. A second study found no difference in cognitive test performance between current and past users of tamoxifen (van Dam et al., 1998). In a third study, a subset of that same cohort of patients underwent cognitive testing two years later (Schagen et al., 2002). No significant differences in risk for cognitive impairment were observed between patients who had completed treatment and those who were still receiving tamoxifen. A large randomized trial is under way comparing the effects of tamoxifen and raloxifene on a variety of outcomes, including cognitive performance, in healthy women at increased risk for breast cancer (Vogel et al., 2002).

Two trials investigated the influence of raloxifene on subjective memory complaints. One compared raloxifene and continuous combined HT in a six-month randomized clinical trial involving 1,008 healthy postmenopausal women (Voss et al., 2002). Women in the HT group reported significantly greater mean improvement in memory and attention but worsened mood compared with the raloxifene group. By contrast, a similar clinical study in 398 healthy, asymptomatic postmenopausal women found no differences in cognitive complaints between groups of women randomly assigned to raloxifene, 60 or 150 mg/day, conjugated equine estrogens (0.625 mg/day), or placebo for 12 months (Strickler et al., 2000).

Two trials of raloxifene have included cognitive outcomes. One small trial concluded that raloxifene had no consistent effect on cognitive function when compared with placebo over 12 months in 143 postmenopausal women (Nickelsen et al., 1999). A large randomized trial of raloxifene in osteoporotic postmenopausal women was recently completed. This trial, the Multiple Outcomes of Raloxifene Evaluation (MORE), evaluated 7,478 women who received either raloxifene (60 or 120 mg/day) or placebo for three years by testing performance on cognitive tests. Mean cognitive scores improved slightly over the three years and were similar in the treatment groups at each visit. Compared to the placebo group, women assigned to raloxifene had a slightly lower risk of developing cognitive decline on an attention test and a verbal memory test, but not on the other four tests (Yaffe et al., 2001). Among women at greater risk for cognitive decline (>70 years old), those assigned to raloxifene performed better compared to placebo recipients on attention and verbal memory tests, but not on the other tests. Reported hot flushes did not influence cognitive test scores or the effect of treatment on test performance ($P \geq 0.3$). Thus, raloxifene treatment for three years did not affect overall cognitive scores in post-menopausal women; however, it may lower the risk of decline in attention and memory domains.

As part of the MORE trial, an ancillary study was conducted to determine the incidence of dementia, including AD, and mild cognitive impairment (MCI) using standardized assessment and an evaluation similar to that used in WHIMS. The goal of the study was to determine whether raloxifene treatment influenced the risk of developing dementia and MCI. After four years of treatment, there was no significant difference between the placebo and the raloxifene (60 mg/day) groups in the risk of developing MCI, AD, dementia from any cause, or any cognitive impairment (dementia and MCI combined). Compared with placebo recipients, women receiving 120 mg/day of raloxifene as a group had a significant, 33 percent lower risk of developing MCI (RR = 0.67, 95% CI: 0.46–0.98; $P = 0.04$), a suggestion of a lower risk of developing AD that was not statistically significant (RR = 0.52, 95% CI: 0.22–1.21; $P = 0.12$), and a 27 percent lower risk of developing any cognitive impairment (RR = 0.73, 95% CI: 0.53–1.01; $P = 0.05$).

Thus, a differential effect of raloxifene on cognitive outcomes by dose was discernible. Although treatment with 120 mg/day of raloxifene reduced the risk of MCI, there was no significant benefit from treatment with the lower dose of 60 mg/day, and the difference in the effect of the two doses was statistically significant. For the treatment of osteoporosis, raloxifene dosages of 60 and 120 mg/day appear to be equally effective (Ettinger et al., 1999). It is possible, however, that higher doses of raloxifene are needed to cross the blood-brain barrier and produce CNS benefits. Furthermore, the raloxifene dose producing maximal increases in hippocampal ChAT activity (3 mg/kg) (Wu et al., 1999) is greater than the dose producing maximal effects on bone (1 mg/kg) in ovariectomized rats (Black et al., 1994).

From the data collected in the MORE trial, it is difficult to determine if raloxifene has an estrogenic, antiestrogenic, or unique effect on the brain. However, given that several observational studies have suggested that estrogen use reduces the risk of developing AD or cognitive impairment (Henderson et al., 1994; Kawas et al., 1997; Tang et al., 1996; Yaffe, Haan, et al., 2000), it is most likely that raloxifene has an estrogenic effect in the CNS (Barkhem et al., 1998). On the other hand, given the recent result from WHIMS indicating an increased risk of developing dementia with estrogen and progestin (Shumaker et al., 2003), it is possible that the reduction in risk of cognitive impairment with raloxifene is due to an antiestrogen effect. Another possible explanation for the differences between our results and those of WHIMS may be related to cardiovascular disease. Unlike estrogen (Shumaker et al., 2003), raloxifene use is not associated with an increase in stroke and other cardiovascular outcomes that may mediate cognitive impairment (Barrett-Connor et al., 2002). Additional trials of raloxifene and other SERMs for the prevention of cognitive impairment and AD, especially in women at high risk, should be conducted to confirm these results.

SERMs and Brain Function in Women

Neuroimaging techniques such as positron emission tomography (PET) and functional magnetic resonance imaging (fMRI) provide insights into the neural targets of SERMs in humans. For example, the influence of tamoxifen and estrogen on brain function and structure was investigated in an observational study involving three groups of postmenopausal women (mean age, 66 years)— 10 breast cancer patients receiving tamoxifen (5 of whom had received radiation treatment, but none had had chemotherapy), 15 healthy current users of HT (ERT+ group), and 15 healthy control subjects who were not using HT (ERT− group) (Eberling et al., 2004). Neuroimaging methods included PET with [18F]fluorodeoxyglucose (FDG), a glucose ligand, to measure regional glucose metabolism during rest, and volumetric MRI to measure hippocampal volume. Cognitive assessments performed in conjunction with the neuroimaging assessments revealed a decrease in semantic memory (object naming) among tamoxifen users compared with the other two groups combined, but no difference on measures of attention span, pattern recognition, or depressive symptoms. Compared with the ERT− group, tamoxifen users showed significant decreases in metabolism in the bilateral superior and medial frontal gyri and left postcentral gyrus. Compared with the ERT+ group, tamoxifen users showed decreases in the left superior frontal gyrus, left and right middle frontal gyrus, and right medial frontal gyrus. Thus, tamoxifen use was associated with decreased frontal lobe metabolism in tamoxifen users compared with both other groups. A region-of-interest analysis focusing on dorsolateral and orbital frontal cortex showed a trend toward lower metabolic rates in right and left orbital frontal cortex. The hippocampal volumes of tamoxifen users were intermediate between those of the HT users and those of nonusers but did not differ significantly from the volume of either group. A post hoc analysis that excluded an outlier revealed lower volume in tamoxifen users than in the ERT+ group. In general, these findings point to possible detrimental effects of tamoxifen on frontal lobe function and hippocampal volume in breast cancer patients.

Proton magnetic resonance spectroscopy, an imaging technique used to assay biochemical markers associated with brain injury, was used in an observational study in three groups of elderly women (mean age, 71 years): ERT+, ERT−, and tamoxifen (Ernst et al., 2002). The results showed significantly lower concentrations of myo-inosit (MI), a glial marker, in the tamoxifen and ERT+ groups compared with the ERT− group. In the light of evidence that MI concentrations increase with aging, this finding was interpreted as indicating a possible beneficial effect of both ERT+ and tamoxifen. The duration of tamoxifen treatment was negatively related to MI concentrations in the basal ganglia and hippocampus. No differences between groups in other biomarkers, including choline-containing compounds (CO) associated with cell membrane metabolism, were detected. The authors interpreted the lack of a difference in these markers as suggesting that tamoxifen, particularly long-term tamoxifen, may not be neurotoxic. However, the interpretation and significance of these findings are unclear, because the study involved only 16 breast cancer patients, and decreased MI levels have been associated with cerebral insults (Ganz et al., 2002). Moreover, the reliability of these findings is unclear, because changes in CO have been reported in HT users compared with nonusers (Robertson et al., 2001).

fMRI was used to measure brain activation during visual encoding and recognition in a three-month, placebo-controlled trial of raloxifene (60 mg/day) (Neele et al., 2001). Postmenopausal women (mean age 66) studied 10 emotionally neutral nature scenes under instructions to remember them for later. Subsequently, brain images were acquired during an encoding task as they viewed those 10 scenes and an additional 60 novel scenes, with instructions to remember them for later. The recognition task took place outside the scanner. A simple photic stimulation task involving alternating flashes of light and darkness served as a control task. No significant group differences were observed on the recognition task. However, raloxifene significantly increased activation in the right superior frontal lobe, right parietal lobe, and right precuneus while decreasing activation in the left parahippocampal gyrus and left lingual gyrus. These data suggest that raloxifene alters brain activation during encoding of visual scenes. It is unclear whether this pattern is one of benefit or detriment.

In an earlier PET study, HT had a similar effect on the parahippocampal gyrus and improved memory on both visual and verbal memory tasks (Resnick et al., 1998). In the light of findings from MORE suggesting a potential beneficial effect of raloxifene on memory (Yaffe et al., 2001) and basic science studies showing that raloxifene targets the hippocampus, these neuroimaging findings suggest that raloxifene might enhance hippocampal function.

Alternative Substances to Treat Vasomotor Symptoms of Menopause

Vitamin E, evening primrose, soy isoflavones, *dong quai,* red clover, naloxone, propranolol, ginseng, yam cream, and Chinese medicinal herbs have been used for treating vasomotor symptoms but have not been found to work well, if at all (Kirschstein, 2003). The frequency of hot flushes can be reduced by clonidine and methyldopa, but these medications can cause dizziness and dry mouth. Currently, venlafaxine is the best-studied antidepressant available and has demonstrated efficacy in the treatment of vasomotor symptoms. Other available agents that have not been adequately studied include SERMs, SSRIs, mirtazapine, gabapentin, chasteberry, and black cohosh. Other modalities to investigate include meditation, acupuncture, hypnosis, biofeedback, deep breathing exercises, and increased exercise; smoking cessation; avoidance of spicy food, caffeine, and alcohol; wearing layered clothing; and maintaining a low ambient temperature (Kirschstein, 2003).

Conclusions

Plausible biological mechanisms might account for a beneficial effect of ET on cognition and dementia, and many observational studies have concluded that ET might prevent dementia, including AD. The WHIMS trial, however, found that HT increased the risk of developing dementia. Given this discrepancy, more research is needed to determine the role of estrogen in cognitive aging. In particular, the neutral and possibly beneficial role of raloxifene on cognitive function overall, and the preliminary data from MORE suggesting a reduction in the risk of cognitive impairment with raloxifene, support additional research on raloxifene and other SERMs. Additional investigation is needed to better understand how genetic polymorphisms regulating sex steroid hormone metabolism and receptor expression may influence cognition. An important broader consideration is whether there are genetic factors in sex hormone pathways that modulate cognitive decline and the response to endogenous steroids on cognition.

REFERENCES

Albagha OM, McGuigan FE, Reid DM, et al. 2001. Estrogen receptor alpha gene polymorphisms and bone mineral density: haplotype analysis in women from the United Kingdom. J Bone Miner Res 16:128–34.

Anderson TI, Wooster R, Laake K, et al. 1997. Screening for ESR mutations in breast and ovarian cancer patients. Hum Mutat 9:531–36.

Barkhem T, Carlsson B, Nilsson Y, et al. 1998. Differential response of estrogen receptor α and estrogen receptor β to partial estrogen agonists/antagonists. Mol Pharmacol 54:105–12.

Barrett-Connor E, Grady D, Sashegyi A, et al. 2002. Raloxifene and cardiovascular events in osteoporotic postmenopausal women: four-year results from the MORE (Multiple Outcomes of Raloxifene Evaluation) randomized trial. JAMA 287:847–57.

Bethea CL, Mirkes SJ, Su A, et al. 2002. Effects of oral estrogen, raloxifene and arzoxifene on gene expression in serotonin neurons of macaques. Psychoneuroendocrinology 27:431–45.

Black LJ, Sato M, Rowley ER, et al. 1994. Raloxifene (LY139481 HCI) prevents bone loss and reduces serum cholesterol without causing uterine hypertrophy in ovariectomized rats. J Clin Invest 93:63–69.

Brandi ML, Becherini L, Gennari L, et al. 1999. Association of the estrogen receptor alpha gene polymorphisms with sporadic Alzheimer's disease. Biochem Biophys Res Commun 265:335–38.

Brookmeyer R, Gray S, Kawas C. 1998. Projections of Alzheimer's disease in the United States and the public health impact of delaying disease onset. Am J Public Health 88:1337–42.

Callier S, Morissette M, Grandbois M, et al. 2001. Neuroprotective properties of 17β-estradiol, progesterone, and raloxifene in MPTP C57Bl/6 mice. Synapse 41:131–38.

Cyr M, Landry M, Di Paolo T. 2000. Modulation by estrogen-receptor directed drugs of 5-hydroxytryptamine-2A receptors in rat brain. Neuropsychopharmacology 23:69–78.

Cyr M, Morissette M, Landry M, et al. 2001. Estrogenic activity of tamoxifen and raloxifene on rat brain AMPA receptors. Neuroreport 12:535–39.

Cyr M, Thibault C, Morissette M, et al. 2001. Estrogen-like activity of tamoxifen and raloxifene on NMDA receptor binding and expression of its subunits in rat brain. Neuropsychopharmacology 25:242–57.

Deng HW, Li J, Li JL, et al. 1999. Association of VDR and estrogen receptor genotypes with bone mass in postmenopausal Caucasian women: different conclusions with different analyses and the implications. Osteoporosis Int 9:499–507.

Draper MW, Flowers DE, Huster WJ, et al. 1996. A controlled trial of raloxifene (LY139481) HCl: impact on bone turnover and serum lipid profile in healthy postmenopausal women. J Bone Miner Res 11:835–42.

Duman RS, Heninger GR, Nestler EJ. 1997. A molecular and cellular theory of depression. Arch Gen Psychiatry 54:597–606.

Eberling JL, Wu C, Tong-Turnbeaugh R, et al. 2004. Estrogen- and tamoxifen-associated effects on brain structure and function. Neuroimage 2:364–71.

Ernst T, Chang L, Cooray D, et al. 2002. The effects of tamoxifen and estrogen on brain metabolism in elderly women. J Natl Cancer Inst 94:592–97.

Ettinger B, Black DM, Mitlak BH, et al. 1999. Reduction of vertebral fracture risk in postmenopausal women with osteoporosis treated with raloxifene: results from a 3-year randomized clinical trial. Multiple Outcomes of Raloxifene Evaluation (MORE) Investigators. JAMA 282:637–45.

Evans DA. 1990. Estimated prevalence of Alzheimer's disease in the United States. Milbank Q 68:267–89.

Farrer LA, Cupples LA, Haines JL, et al. 1997. Effects of age, sex, and ethnicity on the association between apolipoprotein E genotype and Alzheimer disease: a meta-analysis. APOE and Alzheimer Disease Meta-Analysis Consortium. JAMA 278:1349–56.

Fugger HN, Foster TC, Gustafsson J, et al. 2000. Novel effects of estradiol and estrogen receptor alpha and beta on cognitive function. Brain Res 883:258–64.

Ganz PA, Castellon SA, Silverman DHS. 2002. Estrogen, tamoxifen, and the brain. J Natl Cancer Inst 94:547–49.

Georgiou I, Syrrou M, Bouba I, et al. 1999. Association of estrogen receptor gene polymorphisms with endometriosis. Fertil Steril 72:164–66.

Grandbois M, Morissette M, Callier S, et al. 2000. Ovarian steroids and raloxifene prevent MPTP-induced dopamine depletion in mice. Neuroreport 11:343–46.

Harris HA, Albert LM, Leathurby Y, et al. 2003. Evaluation of an estrogen receptor-β agonist in animal models of human disease. Endocrinology 144:4241–49.

Henderson VW, Paganini-Hill HA, Emanuel CK, et al. 1994. Estrogen replacement therapy in older women: comparisons between Alzheimer's disease cases and nondemented control subjects. Arch Neurol 51:896–900.

Herrington DM, Howard TD, Hawkins GA, et al. 2002. Estrogen-receptor polymorphisms and effects of estrogen replacement on high-density lipoprotein cholesterol in women with coronary disease. N Engl J Med 346:967–74.

Isoe-Wada K, Maeda M, Yong J, et al. 1999. Positive association between an estrogen receptor gene polymorphism and Parkinson's disease with dementia. Eur J Neurol 6:431–35.

Jensen EV, Jordan VC. 2003. The estrogen receptor: a model for molecular medicine. Clin Cancer Res 9:1980–89.

Jones KA, Kadonaga JT. 2000. Exploring the transcription-chromatin interface. Genes Dev 14:1992–96.

Jordan VC. 2003. Antiestrogens and selective estrogen receptor modulators as multifunctional medicines. 1. Receptor interactions. J Med Chem 46:883–908.

Katzenellenbogen BS, Katzenellenbogen JA. 2000. Estrogen receptor transcription and transactivation: estrogen receptor alpha and estrogen receptor beta: regulation by selective estrogen receptor modulators and importance in breast cancer. Breast Cancer Res 2:335–44.

Kawas C, Resnick S, Morrison A, et al. 1997. A prospective study of estrogen replacement therapy and the risk of developing Alzheimer's disease: the Baltimore Longitudinal Study of Aging. Neurology 48:1517–21.

Kirschstein R. 2003. Menopausal hormone therapy: summary of a scientific workshop. Ann Intern Med 138:361–64.

Kuiper GGJM, Carlsson B, Grandien K, et al. 1997. Comparison of the ligand binding specificity and transcript tissue distribution of estrogen receptors α and β. Endocrinology 138:863–70.

Labrie F, El-Alfy M, Berger L, et al. 2003. The combination of a novel selective estrogen receptor modulator with an estrogen protects the mammary gland and uterus in a rodent model: the future of postmenopausal women's health? Endocrinology 144:4700–706.

Lacreuse A, Wilson ME, Herndon JG. 2002. Estradiol, but not raloxifene, improves aspects of spatial working memory in aged ovariectomized rhesus monkeys. Neurobiol Aging 23:589–600.

Lambert JC, Harris JM, Mann D, et al. 2001. Are the estrogen receptors involved in Alzheimer's disease? Neurosci Lett 306:193–97.

Launer LJ, Andersen K, Dewey ME, et al. 1999. Rates and risk factors for dementia and Alzheimer's disease: results from EURODEM pooled analyses. EURODEM Incidence Research Group and Work Groups. European Studies of Dementia. Neurology 52:78–84.

Lei DL, Long JM, Hengemihle J, et al. 2003. Effects of estrogen and raloxifene on neuroglia number and morphology in the hippocampus of aged female mice. Neuroscience 121:659–66.

Lonard DM, Smith CL. 2002. Molecular perspectives on selective estrogen receptor modulators (SERMs): progress in understanding their tissue-specific agonist and antagonist actions. Steroids 67:15–24.

Maruyama H, Toji H, Harrington CR, et al. 2000. Lack of an association of estrogen receptor alpha gene polymorphisms and transcriptional activity with Alzheimer disease. Arch Neurol 57:236–40.

Mattila KM, Axelman K, Rinne JO, et al. 2000. Interaction between estrogen receptor 1 and the epsilon4 allele of apolipoprotein E increases the risk of familial Alzheimer's disease in women. Neurosci Lett 282:45–48.

McDonnell DP, Norris JD. 2002. Connections and regulation of the human estrogen receptor. Science 296:1642–44.

McEwen BS. 1999. Clinical review 108: The molecular and neuroanatomical basis for estrogen effects in the central nervous system. J Clin Endocrinol Metab 84:1790–97.

McEwen BS. 2002. Estrogen actions throughout the brain. Recent Prog Horm Res 57:357–84.

McKenna NJ, O'Malley BW. 2002. Minireview: nuclear receptor coactivators: an update. Endocrinology 143:2461–65.

Meisel RL, Dohanich GP, McEwen BS, et al. 1987. Antagonism of sexual behavior in female rats by ventromedial hypothalamic implants of antiestrogen. Neuroendocrinology 45:201–7.

Murer MG, Yan Q, Raisman-Vozari R. 2001. Brain-derived neurotrophic factor in the control human brain, and in Alzheimer's disease and Parkinson's disease. Prog Neurobiol 63:71–124.

Murphy DD, Cole NB, Segal M. 1998. Brain-derived neurotrophic factor mediates estradiol-induced dendritic spine formation in hippocampal neurons. Proc Natl Acad Sci USA 95:11412–17.

Nagy L, Kao HY, Chakravarti D, et al. 1997. Nuclear receptor repression mediated by a complex containing SMRT, mSin3A, and histone deacetylase. Cell 89:373–80.

Neele SJ, Rombouts SA, Bierlaagh MA, et al. 2001. Raloxifene affects brain activation patterns in postmenopausal women during visual encoding. J Clin Endocrinol Metab 86:1422–24.

Nickelsen T, Lufkin EG, Riggs BL, et al. 1999. Raloxifene hydrochloride, a selective estrogen receptor modulator: safety assessment of effects on cognitive function and mood in postmenopausal women. Psychoneuroendocrinology 24:115–28.

Nilsen J, Mor G, Naftolin F. 1998. Raloxifene induces neurite outgrowth in estrogen receptor positive PC12 cells. Menopause 5:211–16.

Nystedt M, Berglund G, Bolund C, et al. 2003. Side effects of adjuvant endocrine treatment in premenopausal breast cancer patients: a prospective randomized study. J Clin Oncol 21:1836–44.

O'Neill K, Chen S, Brinton RD. 2004. Impact of the selective estrogen receptor modulator, raloxifene, on neuronal survival and outgrowth following toxic insults associated with aging and Alzheimer's disease. Exp Neurol 185:63–80.

Osterlund MK, Grandien K, Keller E, et al. 2000. The human brain has distinct regional expression patterns of estrogen receptor alpha mRNA isoforms derived from alternative promoters. J Neurochem 75:1390–97.

Paech K, Webb P, Kuiper GGJM, et al. 1997. Differential ligand activation of estrogen receptors ERα and ERβ at AP1 sites. Science 277:1508–10.

Paganini-Hill A, Clark LJ. 2001. Preliminary assessment of cognitive function in breast cancer patients treated with tamoxifen. Breast Cancer Res Treat 64:165–76.

Panickar KS, Guan G, King MA, et al. 1997. 17β-Estradiol attenuates CREB decline in the rat hippocampus following seizure. J Neurobiol 33:961–67.

Pettersson K, Delaunay F, Gustafsson J-A. 2000. Estrogen receptor β acts as a dominant regulator of estrogen signaling. Oncogene 19:4970–78.

Pike ACW, Brzozowski AM, Hubbard RE, et al. 1999. Structure of the ligand-binding domain of oestrogen receptor beta in the presence of a partial agonist and a full antagonist. EMBO J 18:4608–18.

Resnick SM, Maki PM, Golski S, et al. 1998. Estrogen effects on PET cerebral blood flow and neuropsychological performance. Horm Behav 34:171–82.

Resnick SM, Metter EJ, Zonderman AB. 1997. Estrogen replacement therapy and longitudinal decline in visual memory: a possible protective effect? Neurology 49:1491–97.

Robertson DM, van Amelsvoort T, Daly E, et al. 2001. Effects of estrogen replacement therapy on human brain aging: an in vivo ¹H MRS study. Neurol 57:2114–17.

Rubinow DR, Schmidt PJ, Roca CA, et al. 2002. Gonadal hormones and behavior in women: concentrations vs. context. In Hormones, Brain and Behavior, ed. DW Pfaff, AP Arnold, AM Etgen, et al., 5:37–73. San Diego: Academic Press.

Savaskan E, Olivieri G, Meier F, et al. 2001. Hippocampal estrogen beta-receptor immunoreactivity is increased in Alzheimer's disease. Brain Res 908:113–19.

Schagen SB, Muller MJ, Boogerd W, et al. 2002. Late effects of adjuvant chemotherapy on cognitive function: a follow-up study in breast cancer patients. Ann Oncol 13: 1387–97.

Schagen SB, van Dam FS, Muller MJ, et al. 1999. Cognitive deficits after postoperative adjuvant chemotherapy for breast carcinoma. Cancer 85:640–50.

Shang Y, Brown M. 2002. Molecular determinants for the tissue specificity of SERMs. Science 295:2465–68.

Sherwin BB. 1988. Estrogen and/or androgen replacement therapy and cognitive functioning in surgically menopausal women. Psychoneuroendocrinology 13:345–57.

Shughrue PJ, Lane MV, Merchenthaler I. 1997. Regulation of progesterone receptor messenger ribonucleic acid in the rat medial preoptic nucleus by estrogenic and antiestrogenic compounds: an in situ hybridization study. Endocrinology 138:5476–84.

Shumaker SA, Legault C, Kuller L, et al. 2004. Conjugated equine estrogens and incidence of probable dementia and mild cognitive impairment in postmenopausal women: Women's Health Initiative Memory Study. JAMA 291:2947–58.

Shumaker SA, Legault C, Rapp SR, et al. 2003. Estrogen plus progestin and the incidence of dementia and mild cognitive impairment in postmenopausal women: the Women's Health Initiative Memory Study: a randomized controlled trial. JAMA 289:2651–62.

Singh M, Meyer EM, Millard WJ, et al. 1994. Ovarian steroid deprivation results in a reversible learning impairment and compromised cholinergic function in female Sprague-Dawley rats. Brain Res 644:305–12.

Singh M, Meyer EM, Simpkins JW. 1995. The effect of ovariectomy and estradiol replacement on brain-derived neurotrophic factor messenger ribonucleic acid expression in cortical and hippocampal brain regions of female Sprague-Dawley rats. Endocrinology 136:2320–24.

Smith CL, O'Malley BW. 2004. Coregulator function: a key to understanding tissue specificity of selective receptor modulators. Endocr Rev 25:45–71.

Sohrabji F, Greene LA, Miranda RC, et al. 1994. Reciprocal regulation of estrogen and NGF receptors by their ligands in PC12 cells. J Neurobiol 25:974–88.

Sohrabji F, Miranda RC, Toran-Allerand CD. 1994. Estrogen differentially regulates estrogen and nerve growth factor receptor mRNAs in adult sensory neurons. J Neurosci 14:459–71.

Srivastava RA, Srivastava N, Averna M, et al. 1997. Estrogen up-regulates apolipoprotein E (ApoE) gene expression by increasing ApoE mRNA in the translating pool via the estrogen receptor alpha-mediated pathway. J Biol Chem 272:33360–66.

Stone DJ, Rozovsky I, Morgan TE, et al. 1998. Increased synaptic sprouting in response to estrogen via an apolipoprotein E–dependent mechanism: implications for Alzheimer's disease. J Neurosci 18:3180–85.

Strickler R, Stovall DW, Merritt D, et al. 2000. Raloxifene and estrogen effects on quality of life in healthy postmenopausal women: a placebo-controlled randomized trial. Obstet Gynecol 96:359–65.

Tang MX, Jacobs D, Stern Y, et al. 1996. Effect of oestrogen during menopause on risk and age at onset of Alzheimer's disease. Lancet 348:429–32.

Tsai M-J, O'Malley BW. 1994. Molecular mechanisms of action of steroid/thyroid receptor superfamily members. Annu Rev Biochem 63:451–86.

Tully T, Bourtchouladze R, Scott R, et al. 2003. Targeting the CREB pathway for memory enhancers. Nat Rev Drug Discov 2:267–77.

van Dam FS, Schagen SB, Muller MJ, et al. 1998. Impairment of cognitive function in women receiving adjuvant treatment for high-risk breast cancer: high-dose versus standard-dose chemotherapy. J Natl Cancer Inst 90:210–18.

Vogel VG, Costantino JP, Wickerham DL, et al. 2002. The study of tamoxifen and raloxifene: preliminary enrollment data from a randomized breast cancer risk reduction trial. Clin Breast Cancer 3:153–59.

Voss S, Quail D, Dawson A, et al. 2002. A randomised, double-blind trial comparing raloxifene HCl and continuous combined hormone replacement therapy in postmenopausal women: effects on compliance and quality of life. Br J Obstet Gynaecol 109:874–85.

Webb P, Lopez GN, Uht RM, et al. 1995. Tamoxifen activation of the estrogen receptor/AP-1 pathway: potential origin for the cell-specific estrogen-like effects of antiestrogens. Mol Endocrinol 9:443–56.

Wu X, Glinn MA, Ostrowski NL, et al. 1999. Raloxifene and estradiol benzoate both fully restore hippocampal choline acetyltransferase activity in ovariectomized rats. Brain Res 847:98–104.

Xu H, Gouras GK, Greenfield JP, et al. 1998. Estrogen reduces neuronal generation of Alzheimer beta-amyloid peptides. Nat Med 4:447–51.

Yaffe K, Haan M, Byers A, et al. 2000. Estrogen use, APOE, and cognitive decline: evidence of gene-environment interaction. Neurology 54:1949–54.

Yaffe K, Krueger K, Sarkar S, et al. 2001. Cognitive function in postmenopausal women treated with raloxifene. N Engl J Med 344:1207–13.

Yaffe K, Lui L-Y, Grady D, et al. 2000. Cognitive decline in women in relation to non-protein-bound oestradiol concentrations. Lancet 356:708–12.

Yaffe K, Lui L-Y, Grady D, et al. 2002. Estrogen receptor I polymorphisms and risk of cognitive impairment in older women. Biol Psychiatry 51:677–82.

Yang C, Edsall R Jr, Harris HA, et al. 2004. ERβ ligands. Part 2. Synthesis and structure-activity relationships of a series of 4-hydroxy-biphenyl-carbaldehyde oxime derivatives. Bioorg Med Chem 12:2553–70.

Zhou W, Koldzic-Zivanovic N, Clarke CH, et al. 2002. Selective estrogen receptor modulator effects in the rat brain. Neuroendocrinology 75:24–33.

Zhou Y, Watters JJ, Dorsa DM. 1996. Estrogen rapidly induces the phosphorylation of the cAMP response element binding protein in rat brain. Endocrinology 137:2163–66.

Conclusion

NATALIE L. RASGON, M.D., Ph.D.

"To Treat or Not to Treat, That Is the Question"

The long-term effects of available hormone treatments remain to be determined, as the field is still in the process of integrating the data. Evidence from basic research supports the neuroprotective effects of hormone therapy (HT) in the central nervous system, yet data in humans are less clear. Several issues regarding the use of hormones as neuroprotective agents have emerged from the preclinical data obtained in studies on humans. Although observational studies suggested that estrogen therapy (ET) decreased the risk for dementia in aging women, randomized trials, most notably the Women's Health Initiative Memory Study, have suggested the opposite. Similarly, observational studies have long upheld the notion of improved cognitive performance in women with dementia who are treated with HT, but randomized studies have narrowed the scope of influence to selective (verbal) memory domains, and even those effects are short-lived at best, according to current knowledge.

Discrepancies among clinical studies are numerous, many reflecting the use of different instruments, populations, and study designs. Still in need of explanation are the observations that women have twice the risk of developing Alzheimer disease (AD) as men and that ET clearly enhances verbal memory in acutely surgically menopausal women. Other questions of pressing interest include which specific subpopulations of women will benefit from ET, the type of estrogen preparation to use, the mode of administration, and the type of progestin that should be added, if any.

Implications for Future Research

After age 65, the risk for AD increases exponentially, and projections based on demographics suggest as much as a fivefold increase in the U.S. population with this disease by 2030 (Kirschstein, 2003). Observational studies suggest that postmenopausal women who receive estrogen have a 50 percent reduction in risk for AD, and these findings are supported by in vitro studies of neuronal cell responses to estrogen in cell culture. A number of ongoing controlled clinical trials, including ours at Stanford, are studying women at increased risk for this disease, paying heed to their other estrogen-associated health risks. Other ongoing studies include a tamoxifen trial and a study of a healthy lifestyle approach in the prevention of breast cancer.

Many American women are using alternative therapies today, even though the safety and efficacy of such therapies often are unknown. Several small-scale clinical trials are evaluating the health effects of alternative substances such as phytoestrogens. Future research should focus on the dose levels of alternative HT, routes of administration, and other treatment regimens for women using combination HT to alleviate the vasomotor and genitourinary symptoms of menopause.

Take-Home Message

The decision to initiate or continue HT is a personal one, made by each woman in consultation with her health care provider and taking into consideration current information about the appropriateness of such therapy in relation to the woman's health and expectations. Hormone therapy helps prevent bone loss, but whether that benefit translates into a reduced risk of fractures remains questionable, as quality-of-life data from clinical trials are lacking (Vastag, 2002). In addition, HT must be taken continuously to prevent bone mass loss, not just for 5 to 10 years after menopause, as previously thought (Vastag, 2002).

As is evident from the analyses and discussions in this book, there are no clear answers to the question of whether to treat or not. The one consistent message is that a women's decision to use HT should be a personal decision made in consultation with her health care provider and taking into account current information regarding the risks and benefits of such treatment and the appropriateness of beginning or continuing treatment. Furthermore, the length of treatment should be as short as possible to provide the desired symptom relief.

Despite the lack of clear answers, it is critical that research continue, because the number of women entering the menopausal transition continues to rise. Although the results of the Women's Health Initiative trial are alarming, the data do not point toward total abandonment of HT for women. Future research should help us address the currently unanswered questions regarding safety and efficacy. Much work has been done to ascertain the biological effects of estrogen in the brain, and a narrow window of opportunity exists for the use of ET by certain women in a specific stage of life.

In closing, just as Plato wrote, in the voice of Socrates, "I am the wisest man alive, for I know one thing, and that is that I know nothing," so researchers studying the neuroendocrinology of aging have gained a clearer understanding of how much remains unknown. The next few years of work should result in a better understanding of the molecular genetics of aging and the definition of specific indications for ET and preferred modes of administration.

"The King Is Dead, Long Live the King!"

The question that naturally follows is what agents will succeed or replace ET. Selective estrogen receptor modulators (SERMs) entered the stage in the 1990s, with tamoxiphene being the first of the generation. Although SERMs provide selective modulation of peripheral estrogen receptors in a predictable pattern, the regulation of central estrogen receptors by SERMs has not yet produced consistent responses. There are no clear guidelines in sight, and we ask our readers—many of them women and their physicians—for patience.

REFERENCES

Kirschstein R. 2003. Menopausal hormone therapy: summary of a scientific workshop. Ann Intern Med 138:361–64.

Vastag B. 2002. Hormone replacement therapy falls out of favor with expert committee. JAMA 287:1923–24.

Index